Body Composition Assessment in Children and Adolescents

Medicine and Sport Science

Vol. 44

Series Editors   *J. Borms*, Brussels
                   M. Hebbelinck, Brussels
                   L.J. Micheli, Boston, Mass.

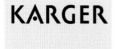

Basel · Freiburg · Paris · London · New York ·
New Delhi · Bangkok · Singapore · Tokyo · Sydney

Body Composition Assessment in Children and Adolescents

Volume Editors   *T. Jürimäe*, Tartu, Estonia
                     A.P. Hills, Brisbane, Australia

26 figures and 50 tables, 2001

KARGER   Basel · Freiburg · Paris · London · New York ·
                 New Delhi · Bangkok · Singapore · Tokyo · Sydney

Medicine and Sport Science

Published on behalf of the International Council of Sport Science and Physical Education
Founder and Editor from 1969 to 1984: E. Jokl†, Lexington, Ky.

••••••••••••••••••••••

Toivo Jürimäe

Faculty of Exercise and Sport Sciences
University of Tartu
18. Ülikooli Street
50090 Tartu (Estonia)

Andrew P. Hills

School of Human Movement Studies
Queensland University of Technology
Kelvin Grove Campus
Victoria Park Road
Kelvin Grove 4059
Brisbane, QLD (Australia)

Library of Congress Cataloging-in-Publication Data

Body composition assessment in children and adolescents / volume editors, T. Jürimäe,
A.P. Hills.
    p.; cm. – (Medicine and sport science; vol. 44)
    Includes bibliographical references and indexes.
    ISBN 3805571313 (hard cover : alk. paper)
    1. Children – Physiology. 2. Teenagers – Physiology. 3. Body
composition – Measurement. I. Jürimäe, T. II. Hills, Andrew P. III. Series.
    [DNLM: 1. Body Composition – Adolescence. 2. Body Composition – Child. 3.
Anthropometry – Adolescence. 4. Anthropometry – Child. QU 100 B6675 2001]
RJ125 .B63 2001
612–dc21

                                                                                00-048745

Bibliographic Indices. This publication is listed in bibliographic services, including Current Contents® and Index Medicus.

Drug Dosage. The authors and the publisher have exerted every effort to ensure that drug selection and dosage set forth in this text are in accord with current recommendations and practice at the time of publication. However, in view of ongoing research, changes in government regulations, and the constant flow of information relating to drug therapy and drug reactions, the reader is urged to check the package insert for each drug for any change in indications and dosage and for added warnings and precautions. This is particularly important when the recommended agent is a new and/or infrequently employed drug.

© Copyright 2001 by S. Karger AG, P.O. Box, CH–4009 Basel (Switzerland)
Printed in Switzerland on acid-free paper by Reinhardt Druck, Basel
ISSN 0254–5020
ISBN 3–8055–7131–3

Contents

Preface

This book has been published because we considered it necessary to present, in a simple publication, details of the methods used in the study of body composition in children with specific examples of the results obtained using some of these approaches. To date, descriptions of methods have often been incomplete in the literature. The following 15 chapters present a range of different aspects of this unique topic ranging from simple anthropometry to the technologically advanced technique of magnetic resonance imaging. This monograph represents what should be considered as the beginning as there is strong evidence to suggest that there is a need to conduct further research on this topic in the future.

Several excellent monographs with an emphasis on body composition assessment have been published in recent years. For example Roche AF, Heymsfield SB, Lohman TG: Human Body Composition. Human Kinetics, Champaign 1996, and Heyward VH, Stolarczyk LM: Applied Body Composition Assessment. Human Kinetics, Champaign 1996. *American Journal of Human Biology* [vol 11/2, 1999] published a special issue concerning body composition. Systematically, international symposia on in vivo body composition studies have been organised, the most recent of which was in Brookhaven National Laboratory, Upton, N.Y., USA in October 1999. However, monographs with a singular focus on the body composition problems in children have been lacking.

Traditional simple approaches in body composition assessment include the use of body stature and body mass as indices of obesity and using the two-component system of estimating fat and lean body mass for describing body composition changes associated with children's growth and development.

The development of better approaches to body composition assessment will lead to an improved understanding of growth and development and the effects of exercise and dietary restriction on body composition. In addition, further research may help provide sound criteria for the validation of new methods of assessment.

Most of the work in the field is descriptive with an emphasis on the effects of growth and maturation and on comparisons of responses to different interventions (for example, diet and exercise) among children, adolescents and adults. Few studies explore the mechanisms of such differences. One of the main reasons for the relatively slow evolution in the knowledge and understanding of child-related issues is ethics. There is little justification, for example, in the use of risky (radioactive markers), painful or potentially extremely uncomfortable procedures (such as hydrostatic weighing), unless these are indicated clinically. There will always be a place for valid and reliable methods which are safe, quick, comfortable and cheap to use with pediatric populations.

In summary, this volume provides details of some new approaches and methods for the measurement of growth and body composition in children and youth of particular relevance to epidemiologists, pediatricians, teachers, coaches and sport specialists.

The editors wish to express their thanks to all of the contributing authors for their support and enthusiasm in the preparation of manuscripts.

Toivo Jürimäe, Tartu
Andrew P. Hills, Brisbane

Jürimäe T, Hills AP (eds): Body Composition Assessment in Children and Adolescents.
Med Sport Sci. Basel, Karger, 2001, vol 44, pp 1–13

....

An Evaluation of the Methodology for the Assessment of Body Composition in Children and Adolescents

Andrew P. Hills, Linda Lyell, Nuala M. Byrne

School of Human Movement Studies, Queensland University of Technology, Queensland, Australia

Technological advances in recent decades have increased the range of opportunities through which the human body can be assessed. However, implementation of the tools available with all populations in the same way may not always be appropriate. Children are not miniature adults. Therefore, while the needs of children and adolescents may be similar to those of adults in many ways, it is important always to be mindful of the differences that exist. This is particularly the case when assessing body composition of individuals of varying ages, ethnic backgrounds, and health status.

Body composition refers to the characteristic size and distribution of the component parts of total body weight (BW). Body composition analysis involves subdividing body weight into two or more compartments according to elemental, chemical, anatomical, or fluid components [1, 2]. The assessment of body composition has traditionally been based on the two-compartment model in which the body is divided into fat mass (FM) and fat-free mass (FFM) [3, 4, 5]. Therefore,

$$FM + FFM = BW.$$

With the utilisation of a range of technologies in body composition assessment, multi-compartmental models have gained more widespread use [6, 7], most commonly incorporating the following levels: total body water (TBW) encompassing extracellular (ECW) and intracellular (ICW) water, fat mass, bone mineral (BM) and protein (P):

$$TBW (ECW + ICW) + FM + BM + P = BW.$$

A well recognised assumption of the two-compartment model, is that the constituents of the FM and FFM compartments have constant densities (0.900 and 1.100 kg/l, respectively) [4, 8]. As outlined by Classey et al. [9], this model further assumes that the relative amounts of the three major components of the FFM (aqueous, mineral, and protein) are known, additive and constant in all individuals. Consequently, methods based on the two-compartmental model are limited when used on individuals who differ from the reference population in bone mineralisation or hydration of their FFM. For example, children have more body water and relatively less BM compared with adults [10]. The chemical composition of the FFM varies throughout childhood and adolescence until values similar to those of adults are achieved around the ages of 17–20 years. Therefore, the relative body fat of children will be overestimated using the traditional two-compartment model. Reilly [11] reported that 'the FFM of children has lower density, lower mineralisation, higher water content, and lower potassium levels' than that of adults and therefore lead to an overestimation of body fat if adult values are utilised in prediction equations.

The only direct way to assess body composition in humans is through the dissection and subsequent analysis of cadavers. Consequently, all other assessment methods are indirect. The limited number of cadaver studies, most of which have been on adults, means that data used to formulate reference standards for body composition in young children are potentially problematic. Many body composition techniques are referred to as doubly indirect, meaning that they rely on another indirect method and are subject to the estimation errors inherent in that and subsequent iterations of the data.

As a result, due to their indirect nature, most of the methods used to measure body composition in humans provide estimations or predictions. Assessment methods range from simple and inexpensive field methods to highly complex and expensive laboratory procedures. Methods can be classified on these two parameters as well as the degree of skill needed by the tester, the type of equipment required, the degree of cooperation expected of the subject, and the validity and reliability of the method. An outline of the various methods available, as well as the respective strengths and weaknesses of each is outlined below. In addition to this evaluation, the appropriateness of each method for the measurement of body composition in children and adolescents is discussed.

The more sophisticated methods of hydrodensitometry, dual energy X-ray absorptiometry (DXA), total body electrical conductivity (TOBEC), total body water (TBW) and total body potassium (TBK) are generally considered reference methods for the assessment of body composition against which other assessment methods are validated. These methods are not readily available for most research projects, particularly when working with large groups of people, as the equipment is expensive and highly specialised. A brief mention is made of the respective strengths and weaknesses of these methodologies which is useful to the practitioner when evaluating prediction equations for use in field methods. The most popular methods for assessment of body composition in the field include bioelectrical impedance analysis (BIA), and anthropometric measures, including skinfolds.

Densitometry

The measurement of whole body density through hydrostatic weighing has traditionally been considered the gold standard in body composition assessment. The method is based on the principle that the weight of the submerged human being is directly related to their body density. Body density represents a combination of the density of body fat and FFM. Whole body density is then used to estimate the contribution of lean and fat tissue using standard equations [12]. This method has several limitations in respect to validity and suitability for use with children. The technique requires a very high degree of subject cooperation, the subject must be able to exhale completely and hold their breath for at least 10 s underwater, and this must be repeated several times. The need to have the head submerged renders the method inappropriate for use with young children.

However, the major shortcomings relate to the assumptions of the hydrostatic method. Fundamentally, the technique assumes a constancy of the density of FFM which is affected by hydration status and contribution of BM to FFM [13]. These components are variable throughout growth and development. Recently, air-displacement plethysmography has been developed (BOD POD body composition system) and has overcome many of the problems associated with underwater weighing such as being submerged underwater [14]. There has been relatively little work undertaken to date using the BOD POD with young children [15].

Total Body Water (TBW)

Measurement of body water by isotope dilution techniques is used to predict the lean body mass using the principle that fat is anhydrous and that lean body mass contains a relatively constant proportion of water. Jensen [12] has indicated that this assumption is not valid and that to compare individuals with a different body composition, extracellular fluid must be measured in addition to TBW. This can be done by measuring the concentration of hydrogen isotopes (deuterium and tritium) in biological fluids (saliva, plasma, urine) [16]. The use of radioactive tracers such as tritium, are contraindicated in research with children. The use of non-radioactive isotopes can make the technique suitable for use in children, however, the cost can be prohibitive and is not likely to be available to all researchers [13]. Measurement of TBW and ECW are useful as body composition assessment techniques however, one needs to be aware of the assumptions commonly made with respect to the water fraction of the FFM [7, 12]. For adults, the water fraction of 73.2% is often employed but this is not constant in adults. Estimates range from approximately 80% in neonates to the adult range of 71–75% at the end of the adolescent period [17]. Higher levels of water content (that is above the assumed values such as 73.2%) will result in an underestimation of percent body fat. Further, protocols need to ensure that no dehydration or superhydration situation exists due to increased exercise or increased fluid intake. Children are renowned for their predisposition to voluntary dehydration.

Total Body Potassium

In the knowledge that potassium is virtually absent in adipose tissue, the measurement of total body potassium (TBK) also permits an estimation of lean body mass. TBK can be measured in two ways, the subject can be placed in a chamber that counts the decay of ^{40}K, a naturally radioactive isotope, or the ^{40}K can be administered to the subject. This option does not require the extensive shielding and sensitive detectors required in a chamber. Based on the radioactivity measured from the counting procedure, TBK can be measured and this is then converted into lean body mass using a factor dependent on the potassium content of FFM. This technique has good accuracy in measuring TBK but the extrapolation to lean body mass may be a source of inaccuracy as the conversion factor needs to be specific to the population being measured. Children have lower potassium levels than adults and levels increase during growth, therefore adult conversion factors are not appropriate. The technique is safe and non-invasive, however the need to be enclosed in a small chamber for a period of time may limit the use of the technique in young children. TBK measurement is a laboratory-based procedure, requires expensive specialised equipment, and the time for measurement can range from 10 up to 150 min [12].

Imaging Techniques

Magnetic Resonance Imaging (MRI)
MRI provides a visual image of adipose tissue and non-fat tissue within the sections of the body scanned. The subject must lie enclosed in a scanner

until sufficient images are obtained to predict total body fat. The weight of fat is then estimated using the known volume and density of fat. It must be noted that the non-fat components of fat (protein and water) will be included in areas of fat and thus the FFM estimate from this technique will be less than that measured using DXA or hydrodensitometry. The benefits of MRI are the ability to measure regional fat distribution and inter-abdominal fat content, and the high degree of accuracy and reliability [18]. Several limitations exist, especially when working with children. The subject must be enclosed in the MRI scanner for a long period of time that may be traumatic, especially for younger children. The method is expensive, time consuming, not accessible to all practitioners and therefore has limited application for work with paediatric populations.

Computed Axial Tomography (CT)

Computed axial tomography uses the same principles as MRI and has similar strengths and weaknesses. Computed axial tomography requires considerable exposure to radiation, and hence is not suitable for use in children.

Absorptiometry (Dual Energy X-Ray Absorptiometry – DXA)

The DXA procedure is based on an analysis of gamma rays emitted from the body in response to a low intensity neutron beam. Lean tissue, bone and fat tissues emit different gamma ray responses from which an estimation of body composition can be made [19]. Elowsson et al. [20] evaluated the accuracy of body composition assessment for children using DXA by comparisons with chemical analysis of pigs. Accurate estimates of BW were made, but not of the composition of the three compartments of BM, FM and FFM. These compartments were either over- or under-estimated depending on the software used. Ogle et al. [21] compared DXA with anthropometric measures of body fat using the equations of Slaughter et al. [22] that account for the chemical immaturity of children. Their findings showed a comparable result for %BF for males, but, however, an overestimation of %BF for females. The researchers recommended that further studies should be conducted to validate the accuracy of DXA measurements in children. Since the publication of Ogle et al. [21], Pintauro et al. [23] conducted a study using pig carcasses to validate the use of DXA in paediatric populations, on which Dezenberg et al. [24] based their research.

According to Heyward and Stolarczyk [25], the advantages of the DXA technique include high reliability, rapidity of measurement, minimal subject cooperation and accounts for differences in bone mineral density of subjects, which is an important consideration in the assessment of children and adolescents. Two disadvantages include the validity of the technique for use in children may need to be further established and the ethical consideration of the necessity for the use of ionising radiation. As yet there are no international standards for dose limits in children, however an appropriate dose range may be <0.1 mSv, which is the lowest risk category of the International Commission on Radiological Protection (ICRP). The dose of the radiation should be based on specific age and sex risk factors and the researchers should assess why the study is required, the type of benefits expected to arise, and the likely harm to the subject.

Heyward [16] stated that estimates of FM depend on the manufacturer, data collection mode and the software version used to assess the data. The technique does not provide reliable information regarding the distribution of body fat, for example in the abdomen [26]. Both Heyward [16] and Reilly [11] agree that the use of DXA as a gold standard is unjustified at this stage.

Electrical Conductance

Total Body Electrical Conductivity (TOBEC)

Assessing body composition using the TOBEC method requires the subject to be placed in a measurement chamber consisting of a large cylindrical coil that generates electrical current at a specific radio frequency. 'This method is based on the principle that a living organism placed in an electromagnetic field perturbs that field. This perturbation is caused by the electrolyte mass within that organism. Since electrolytes reside exclusively in the FFM, it has been possible through proper calibration, to achieve an accurate separation of this body compartment from body fat' [27].

The paediatric TOBEC instruments yield more accurate data than adult instruments as animal carcasses have been used to calibrate the paediatric instrument, whereas indirect methods were used to calibrate the adult versions [27]. This methodology is particularly suited to children as it is non-invasive, and non-threatening, safe as it does not involve the use of radiation, quick and requires minimal cooperation from the subject. The research conducted by Klish [27] indicates a high degree of both reliability and validity of the methodology, however it also may require further research to support these claims as the methodology is relatively new.

Bioelectrical Impedance Analysis (BIA)

The evaluation of body composition using the BIA method involves passing a low-level electrical current through the individual's body and measuring the impedance or opposition to the flow of current. Electrolytes in the body water are excellent conductors of electricity. Assuming a relatively constant hydration of FFM, TBW measures can be used to predict FFM. The body's FFM can then be predicted as the water content of FFM is relatively large. As adipose tissue is a poor conductor of electricity due to its small water content, the resistance in an individual with large amounts of body fat will be higher than that of an individual with a greater percentage of FFM. Research on segmental versus whole-body bioimpedance has shown that the electrical resistance is primarily influenced by the limbs, suggesting that the technique may be relatively insensitive to differences in tissue composition of the trunk [28].

Schaefer et al. [29] compared BIA and skinfold measures of FFM derived from TBK in children with a mean age of 11.8 years. They found far better intra-observer and inter-observer reliability with BIA than that achieved with skinfold measures, however, once these were accounted for, the FFM estimates were similar for BIA and anthropometry. Okasora et al. [30] compared BIA and DXA as methods of body composition assessment in children and found close correlation between %BF, FFM and body fat content. The limitation of this study was that equations used by the researchers were those of Brozek et al. [4]. These equations are widely recognised as inappropriate for use in children as they do not account for the variability of the composition of the FFM in young individuals. Correlation coefficients were also the only statistical analyses used and Reilly [11] states that correlation is not evidence of agreement when validating body composition assessment methods. Bland and Altman plots or an analysis of the size of the prediction error should be utilised to determine if there is agreement between the two measures.

BIA is a reasonable body composition assessment technique in children because measurements are fast, noninvasive, inexpensive, painless, require little subject cooperation, does not require a high level of technical skill and can be used to estimate body composition in obese individuals [25, 29]. BIA accurately predicts %BF in children provided that an appropriate prediction equation is utilised. Heyward and Stolarczyk [25] recommend the equations of Houtkooper et al. [31] for boys and girls 10–19 years old and for children younger than 10, the BIA equations of Lohman [32] or Kushner et al. [33]. These equations were developed using a three-compartment model and have prediction errors of 2.1 kg or less.

The reliability of a method is dependent at least in part on the protocol used in the measurement. A number of factors can influence BIA measurements including the level of hydration of the subject, posture, measurement protocol, environmental and/or skin temperature, age, gender, athletic status, body composition status and ethnic origin. Moreover, the use of BIA to assess changes in an individual over time must ideally control for biological and environmental variables such as hydration status, timing and content of last ingested meal, skin temperature and menstrual cycle [34].

Anthropometry

The widespread use of a systematised approach to the measurement of children and adolescents has resulted in a range of acceptable measurement approaches or standards. Readers are referred to the following sources for descriptions of anthropometric techniques [35–38] and methodological assessment [39].

Anthropometric Indices

Anthropometric measurements can be used to assess body size and proportions as well as total body and regional body composition. Measures include body weight and stature, proportions of body segments, circumferences, skinfolds, skeletal diameters, and segment lengths. Anthropometric indices include BMI and the waist to hip ratio (WHR). Apart from skinfolds, measures are relatively simple, inexpensive and do not require a high degree of technical skill. However, a degree of subject cooperation is required which may present challenges in assessing young children. From a practical perspective, the physical measurement of children presents a range of unique challenges. Crawford [40] has indicated that children may be more curious, more cautious, less patient and less capable of sustaining postural positions required compared with adults.

Potential sources of error in the use of anthropometric methods are the equipment plus technical skill of the tester, subject factors, and the prediction equation selected to estimate body composition. Prediction equations have been published for use in children and use combinations of circumferences and skeletal diameters to predict body density. However, Heyward and Stolarczyk [25] report that the equations developed by Boileau et al. [41] significantly over or underestimated body density in two samples of children. Further, they suggested that these anthropometric equations should not be used to assess body composition in children. These measures are best suited to large-scale epidemiological studies and for clinical purposes.

Body Mass Index (BMI)

BMI is perhaps the most common anthropometric measure used to predict relative overweight. However, the value of the measurement in children and adolescents is regularly questioned. The natural course of growth and maturation in children, plus the individual variability during the same period mean that indices of weight-for-height, including the BMI (W/H^2) are not very good indices of adiposity [42]. In children younger than 15 years of age, BMI is not totally independent of height and thus should be used with caution. Both Schey et al. [43] and Michielutte et al. [44] examined the value of various weight-for-height indices and found that BMI was the most useful. However, in paediatric populations there is a correlation with height that is not noted in adult populations. BMI was found to correlate less strongly with the triceps skinfold measure at younger ages. Both papers concluded by suggesting that practitioners be cautious in using BMI as a measure of adiposity in children and that, if possible, multiple criteria should be used in assessing body composition. Deurenberg et al. [45] stated that BMI could accurately predict body fat percentage using equations however the SEE in children was 4.4%BF which is above the cut-off (3–4%BF) proposed by Reilly [11] to indicate acceptable accuracy. This finding indicates that BMI is useful as a classifying tool in epidemiological studies, but, however, has limited use in body composition assessment.

Skinfolds

Skinfolds are used to estimate the regional fat distribution by determining the ratio of subcutaneous fat on the trunk and extremities. Skinfolds measure the thickness of two layers of skin and the underlying subcutaneous fat using calipers. Use of the technique to derive a percent body fat value assumes that the distribution of fat subcutaneously and internally is similar for all individuals and that there is a relationship between subcutaneous fat and total body fat. This method also assumes that there is a relationship between the sum of skinfolds and body density that is linear for homogeneous samples indicating that a population-specific prediction equation must be used.

Dezenberg et al. [24] recently evaluated the skinfold equations published by Slaughter et al. [22] and Goran et al. [46] for use in children. They concluded that neither of these equations accurately predicted FM in a heterogeneous group of 4- to 11-year-old children. The researchers then developed and cross-validated a new prediction equation which was found to be valid for ethnic and gender sub-groups and a range of up to 30 kg of body fat. This equation is as follows:

$$\text{FM (kg)} = 0.38*\text{body weight} + (0.30*\text{triceps}) + (0.87*\text{gender}) + (0.81*\text{ethnicity}) - 9.42,$$

where gender = 1 for males and 2 for females, and ethnicity = 1 for Caucasians and 2 for African-Americans.

Skinfold measurements have the advantage that they require minimal and relatively inexpensive equipment. The portability of equipment makes field measures relatively simple. The technique is potentially threatening as some children may perceive the calipers to be uncomfortable or even painful, which may minimise the amount of subject cooperation. The technique also requires a high degree of technical skill for the method to be reliable, especially important in longitudinal studies of growth and development. To increase reliability and accuracy the same calipers should be used to assess change in skinfolds. The same side of the body should be used for consistency, and the practitioner should accurately measure the same skinfold sites used in the chosen prediction equation. The subject should not be measured immediately after exercise and the menstrual cycle of young women should be accounted for in repeated measurements.

Near Infra-Red Interactance Method

The near infra-red interactance method is a relatively new field method to estimate body composition. This technique involves the use of a beam of infra-red radiation applied to a selected skinfold site and the measurement of the intensity and pattern of reflected radiation. The resultant optical densities are combined in a densitometrically based equation combined with height, weight and a measure of the subject's activity level. Jensen [12] stated that it would appear unlikely that one could validly extrapolate composition data from a limited subcutaneous depot to the entire body and expect consistent and valid results.

The usefulness of this measure is based on assumptions that according to Heyward and Stolarczyk [25] have not been supported by research. This leads to an overestimation of %BF at the measurement site. As the method is relatively new, limited research has been conducted to develop and validate prediction models. Heyward [16] states that the Futrex-5000™ equations over-estimate %BF of children because they have been calibrated against densitom-etry. Therefore, these equations are not recommended for body composition assessment of children or adolescents. This technique may have application in the future as an appropriate field method because it requires little technical skill, little subject cooperation and minimal equipment, however much more research needs to be conducted before the technique is used as an assessment tool.

Conclusion

Both the DXA and TOBEC methodologies are promising as reference methods for body composition assessment however, both are relatively new and require further validation. These methods have the advantage of being non-invasive, time-efficient and require little subject cooperation. Disadvantages are that both are expensive and require specialised equipment that may only be available to a small number of researchers and practitioners. BIA, skinfolds and anthropometry are the most appropriate for use in the field. The techniques provide satisfactory validity providing the appropriate equations are used for the specific population. The current best prediction equations have been noted in this paper. BIA may hold the advantage over skinfolds as the technique is less invasive, requires less technical skill, has both higher inter- and intra-tester reliability, is quicker and may be easier to administer to young children.

References

1   Heymsfield SB, Masako W: Body composition in humans: Advances in the development of multicompartment chemical models. Nutr Rev 1991;49:97–108.
2   Wang Z, Ma R, Pierson RN, Heymsfield SB: Five-level model: Reconstruction of body weight at atomic, molecular, cellular, and tissue-system levels from neutron activation analysis. Basic Life Sci 1993;60:125–128.
3   Behnke AR, Wilmore JH: Evaluation and Regulation of Body Build and Composition. Englewood Cliffs, Prentice Hall, 1974.
4   Brozek J, Grande F, Anderson JT, Keys A: Densitometric analysis of body composition: Revision of some quantitative assumptions. Ann NY Acad Sci 1963;110:113–140.
5   Siri WE: The gross composition of the body; in Tobias CA, Lawrence JH (eds): Advances in Biological and Medical Physics. New York, Academic Press, 1956, vol 4, pp 239–280.
6   Wells JCK, Fuller NJ, Dewit O, Fewtrell MS, Elia M, Cole TJ: Four-compartment model of body composition in children: Density and hydration of fat-free mass and comparison with simpler models. Am J Clin Nutr 1999;69:904–912.
7   Roemmich JN, Clark PA, Weltman A, Rogol AD: Alterations in growth and body composition during puberty. I. Comparing multicompartment body composition models. J Appl Physiol 1997; 83:927–935.
8   Visser M, Gallagher D, Deurenberg P, Wang J, Pierson RN, Heymsfield SB: Density and fat-free body mass: Relationship with race, age, and level of fatness. Am J Physiol 1997;272:E781–E787.
9   Classey JL, Kanaley JA, Wideman L, Heymsfield SB, Teates CD, Gutgesell ME, Thorner MO, Hartman ML, Weltman A: Validity of methods of body composition assessment in young and older men and women. J Appl Physiol 1999;86:1728–1738.
10 Lohman TG, Boileau RA, Slaughter MH: Body composition in children and youth; in Bioleau RA (ed): Advances in Pediatric Sport Sciences. Champaign, Human Kinetics, 1984, pp 29–57.
11 Reilly JJ: Assessment of body composition in infants and children. Nutrition 1998;14:821–825.
12 Jensen MD: Research techniques for body composition assessment. J Am Diet Assoc 1992;92: 454–460.
13 Lukaski HC: Methods for the assessment of human body composition: Traditional and new. Am J Clin Nutr 1987;46:537–556.
14 Elia M, Ward LC: New techniques in nutritional assessment: Body composition methods. Proc Nutr Soc 1999;58:33.
15 Dewit O, Fuller NJ, Elia M, Wells CJK: Whole-body plethysmography compared with hydrodensitometry for body composition analysis. Proc Nutr Soc 1998;58:59A.
16 Heyward VH: Practical body composition assessment for children, adults and older adults. Int J Sport Nutr 1998;8:285–307.
17 Haschke F: Body composition of adolescent males. II. Body composition of male reference adolescents. Acta Paediatr Scand 1983;307:13–23.
18 Ross R, Shaw KD, Martel Y, de Guise J, Avruch L: Adipose tissue distribution measured by magnetic resonance imaging in obese women. Am J Clin Nutr 1993;57:470–475.
19 Ellis KJ, Shypailo RJ, Pratt JA, Pond WG: Accuracy of dual energy X-ray absorptiometry for body composition measurements in children. Am J Clin Nutr 1994;60:660–665.

20 Elowsson P, Forslund AH, Mallin H, Fuek U, Hansson I, Carlsten J: An evaluation of dual-energy X-ray absorptiometry and underwater carcass analysis in piglets. J Nutr 1998;128:1543–1549.

21 Ogle GD, Allen JR, Humphries IRJ, Lu PW, Briody JN, Morely K, Howman-Giles R, Cowell CT: Body composition assessment by dual energy X-ray absorptiometry in subjects aged 4–26y. Am J Clin Nutr 1995;61:746–753.

22 Slaughter MH, Lohman TG, Boileau RA, Horswill CA, Stillman RJ, Van Loan MD, Bemben DA: Skinfold equations for estimation of body fatness in children and youth. Hum Biol 1988;60:709–723.

23 Pintauro S, Nagy TR, Duthie C, Goran MI: Cross-calibration of fat and lean measurements by dual energy X-ray absorptiometry to pig carcass analysis in the pediatric body weight range. Am J Clin Nutr 1996;63:293–299.

24 Dezenberg C, Nagy T, Gower R, Johnson R, Goran M: Predicting body composition from anthropometry in pre-adolescent children. Int J Obes 1999;23:253–259.

25 Heyward VH, Stolarczyk LM: Applied Body Composition Assessment. Champaign, Human Kinetics, 1996.

26 Garrow J: Clinical assessment of obesity; in: British Nutrition Foundation, Obesity. Oxford, Blackwell Science, 1999, p 19.

27 Klish WJ: Use of TOBEC instrument in the measurement of body composition in children; in Kral JG, Van Itallie TB (eds): Recent Developments in Body Composition Analysis: Methods and Applications. London, Smith-Gordon, 1993, pp 111–120.

28 Zhu F, Schneditz D, Wang Energy, Levin NW: Dynamics of segmental extracellular volumes during changes in body position by bioelectrical impedance. J Appl Physiol 1997;85:497–504.

29 Schaefer F, Georgi M, Zieger A, Scharer K: Usefulness of bioelectric impedance and skinfold measurements in predicting fat-free mass derived from total body potassium in children. Pediatr Res 1994;35:617–624.

30 Okasora K, Takaya R, Tokuda M, Fukunaga Y, Oguni T, Tanaka H, Konishi K, Tamai H: Comparison of bioelectrical impedance analysis and dual energy X-ray absorptiometry for assessment of body composition in children. Pediatr Int 1999;41:121–125.

31 Houtkooper LB, Going SB, Lohman TG, Roche AF, Van Loan M: Bioelectrical impedance estimation of fat-free body mass in children and youth: A cross-validation study. J Appl Physiol 1992;72: 366–373.

32 Lohman TG: Advances in Body Composition Assessment. Current Issues in Exercise Science Series, monogr 3. Champaign, Human Kinetics, 1992.

33 Kushner RF, Schoeller DA, Fjeld CR, Danford L: Is the impedance index (ht^2/R) significant in predicting total body water? Am J Clin Nutr 1992;56:835–839.

34 Hills AP, Byrne NM: Bioelectrical impedance: use and abuse; in Coetsee MF, Van Heerden HJ (eds): Proceedings of the International Council for Physical Activity and Fitness Research, Itala, South Africa, 1997, p 23.

35 Weiner JS, Lourie JA: Practical Human Biology. New York, Academic Press, 1981.

36 Cameron N: The methods of auxological anthropometry; in Falkner F, Tanner JM (eds): Human Growth: A Comprehensive Treatise. New York, Plenum Press, 1986.

37 Lohman TG, Roche AF, Martorell R: Anthropometric Standardisation Reference Manual. Champaign, Human Kinetics, 1988.

38 Ross WD, Marfell-Jones MJ: Kinathropometry; in MacDougall JD, Wenger HA, Green HJ (eds): Physiological Testing of the High-Performance Athlete. Champaign, Human Kinetics, 1991, pp 223–308.

39 Zemel BS, Riley EM, Stallings VA: Evaluation of methodology for nutritional assessment in children: Anthropometry, body composition, and energy expenditure. Ann Rev Nutr 1997;17:211–235.

40 Crawford SM: Anthropometry; in Docherty D (ed): Measurement in Pediatric Exercise Science. Champaign, Human Kinetics, 1996, p 21.

41 Boileau RA, Wilmore JH, Lohman TG, Slaughter MH, Riner WF: Estimation of body density from skinfold thicknesses, body circumferences and skeletal widths in boys aged 8 to 11 years: Comparison of two samples. Hum Biol 1981;53:575–592.

42 Lazarus R, Baur L, Webb K, Blyth F: Adiposity and body mass indices in children: Benn's index and other weight for height indices as measures of adiposity. Int J Obes 1996;20:406–412.

43 Schey H, Michielutte R, Corbett W, Schey H, Ureda J: Weight for height indices as measures of adiposity in children. J Chron Dis 1984;37:397–400.

44 Michielutte R, Diseker R, Corbett W, Schey H, Ureda J: The relationship between weight height indices and the triceps skinfold measure among children age 5 to 12. Am J Publ Hlth 1984;74: 604–606.

45 Deurenberg P, van der Kooy K, Leenan R, Westrate JA, Seidell JC: Sex and age specific population prediction formulas for estimating body composition from bioelectrical impedance: A cross-validation study. Int J Obes 1991;15:17–25.

46 Goran MI, Driscoll P, Johnson R, Nagy TR, Hunter G: Cross-calibration of body composition techniques against dual-energy X-ray absorptiometry in young children. Am J Clin Nutr 1996;63: 299–305.

Andrew P. Hills, PhD, School of Human Movement Studies, Queensland University of Technology, Victoria Park Road, Kelvin Grove, Queensland 4059 (Australia)
Tel. +61 7 3864 3286, Fax +61 7 3864 3980, E-Mail a.hills@qut.edu.au

Jürimäe T, Hills AP (eds): Body Composition Assessment in Children and Adolescents.
Med Sport Sci. Basel, Karger, 2001, vol 44, pp 14–24

··························

Comparison of Arm-to-Leg and Leg-to-Leg (Standing) Bioelectrical Impedance Analysis for the Estimation of Body Composition in 8- to 10-Year-Old Children

Ann V. Rowlands, Roger G. Eston

School of Sport, Health and Exercise Sciences, University of Wales, Bangor, UK

Obesity in adult life is linked with many chronic diseases [1]. Childhood obesity has been shown to increase the risk of obesity in adulthood [2] and has been linked with coronary artery disease risk factors [3]. Although the developed world is perhaps more aware of the risks of increased levels of body fat than ever before, the incidence of obesity is increasing in children [4] and in adults [5]. It is not only pathological cases of obesity that are on the increase. The average child in the 1980s was fatter than the average child 20 years earlier [6]. At the opposite end of the scale there are a small number of children, predominantly girls, who develop eating disorders which can lead to dangerously low levels of body fat [7].

The current focus on health, fitness and fatness in the media has led to the development of a new and easy to use single frequency bioelectrical impedance analysis (BIA) system (Tanita, TBF 105/305, Tanita Corporation, Tokyo, Japan). The system measures impedance from leg-to-leg in the standing position, rather than the widely used arm-to-leg method, with the subject in the supine position. The four electrodes are stainless steel pressure footpads which are mounted on a scale [8]. Hence, all the subject needs to do is stand on the platform in their bare feet. Body mass and leg-to-leg impedance are then measured simultaneously. No skill is required as electrodes do not need to be placed at specific sites on the body.

In a small sample of adults, leg-to-leg BIA measured using the pressure footpads, correlated highly with leg-to-leg BIA measured using traditional gel electrodes (n=9, r=0.99, p<0.001) [8]. However, there was a significant difference between the two impedance values derived (p<0.001). The pressure footpads leg-to-leg impedance reading was approximately 15 Ω higher than the gel electrode leg-to-leg impedance. Correlations between fat-free mass (FFM) (predicted by hydrodensitometry) and stature-corrected impedance (height^2/impedance) were slightly higher for the arm-to-leg method than the leg-to-leg method (r=0.93, p<0.001 cf. r=0.89, p<0.001, n=231). The authors concluded that the leg-to-leg BIA system had performance characteristics similar to the arm-to-leg unit, but there were systematic differences in impedance measured by pressure footpads, compared to gel electrodes. The body composition (fat mass, fat free mass and percent fat) output from the BIA systems was not considered. Presumably, this was because these measurements rely on the accuracy of the built-in regression equation as well as the accuracy of the impedance measurement. However, the validity of the output measure is very important if the system is being used in settings such as health clubs and private homes where there is no access to or desire to use alternative prediction equations.

Systems which allow the prediction of percent fat in children as well as adults are readily available. However, to the authors' knowledge, there are no published papers pertaining to the validity of this technique in children. Arm-to-leg BIA has been validated in children against the criteria of skinfolds [9], hydrodensitometry [10] and total body water [10, 11]. Stature-corrected resistance was found to be an accurate predictor of total body water in 4- to 6-year-old children [11], of FFM in 10- to 14-year-olds (r=0.94, p<0.001, n=94) [10] and in 94 Chinese boys and girls aged 11–17 years (boys r=0.96, p<0.001, n=48, girls r=0.74, p<0.001, n=46) [9].

The criterion measures in the present study were percent fat and FFM predicted by skinfolds. When assessing body composition in children the assumptions of the two component model are violated as the proportion of water and bone mineral content of the FFM change during growth [12], hence a multicomponent approach should be used for assessing FFM in children, such as in the study by Houtkooper et al. [10]. The skinfold prediction equations used in the present study were developed using multicomponent reference measures [13]. In addition, the prediction equation for percent fat was cross-validated by Janz et al. [14] in 55 girls aged between 8 and 17 years. The criterion measure was hydrodensitometry using Lohman's Siri age-adjusted body density equation [12]. The error associated with the prediction (SEE = 3.6%) was within acceptable limits [15]. Janz et al. [14], therefore, concluded that this equation was valid.

The purpose of the present study was to compare impedance measurements and prediction of percent fat in children using a leg-to-leg BIA system and an arm-to-leg BIA system. The criterion measure was percent fat and FFM predicted by skinfolds.

Method

Subjects were 34 Caucasian children (17 boys and 17 girls), ages 8.3–10.8 years [9.5 ± 0.7 (SD) years; mass 31.2 ± 5.0 kg; height 134.4 ± 7.1 cm] from two local primary schools in Bangor, North Wales. Written informed consent was obtained from the children's parents or guardians.

Anthropometric data were recorded in each child's home. Height was measured with a free-standing Seca stadiometer. Leg-to-leg impedance and body mass were measured simultaneously by the Tanita TBF-305 body composition scales (Tanita UK Ltd., Middlesex, UK). This required the subject to stand on the footpads housing the electrodes, ensuring that the front of each foot was in contact with the toe electrode and the rear of each foot in contact with the heel electrode. The footpads were cleaned with alcohol swabs prior to each measurement. Body mass, impedance and the prediction of percent fat were recorded for each child. Arm-to-leg impedance was measured with the subject lying supine using the Bodystat 1500 (Bodystat, Isle of Man, UK). The current electrodes were placed on the dorsal surface of the right hand and right foot at the distal metacarpals and metatarsals, respectively. The detector electrodes were placed next to the ulnar head of the right wrist and between the medial and lateral malleolus of the right ankle. Alcohol swabs were used to clean the sites prior to attachment of the electrodes. Impedance and predicted percent body fat were recorded for each child.

Skinfolds were taken at two sites: triceps (vertical fold midway between the olecranon process and the acromion process) and subscapular (oblique skinfold 1 cm below the inferior angle of the scapula). Each skinfold was measured twice with Holtain skinfold calipers (Crosswell, Crymych, South Wales, UK). If the readings differed by more than 1 mm, a third reading was taken and the mean recorded. The triceps and subscapular skinfold were used to predict percent body fat using the following equations, based on multicomponent models for Caucasian children:

Σ triceps + subscapular
$\quad$ Σ SKF > 35 mm

Boys (all ages)	% fat = 0.783(Σ SKF) + 1.6
Girls (all ages)	% fat = 0.546(Σ SKF) + 9.7

$\quad$ Σ SKF < 35 mm

Pre-pubertal boys	% fat = 1.21(Σ SKF) − 0.008(Σ SKF)^2 − 1.7
Girls (all ages)	% fat = 1.33(Σ SKF) − 0.013(Σ SKF)^2 − 2.5

Slaughter et al. [13].

Data Analysis

Output measures were: percent fat predicted from the Tanita (leg-to-leg BIA), the Bodystat (arm-to-leg BIA) and skinfolds; FFM predicted from skinfolds; BMI (body mass index, kg/m^2); impedance measured by the Tanita and the Bodystat (Ω); stature-corrected impedance (height^2/impedance) for both the Tanita and the Bodystat. Descriptive statistics were calculated for all variables.

Differences between the impedance values from arm-to-leg and from leg-to-leg were investigated using a 2-way mixed model ANOVA. Independent variables were measurement method (Bodystat, Tanita) and gender (boys, girls) with repeated measures on measurement method. Differences between the prediction of percent body fat from each method were also investigated using a 2-way mixed model ANOVA. Independent variables were prediction method (skinfolds, Bodystat, Tanita) and gender (boys, girls) with repeated measures on prediction method. Tukey's post-hoc tests were used where appropriate.

Pearson product moment correlations were used to assess the relationships between: the impedance measurements from both machines; skinfold predicted FFM with stature-corrected impedance; percent fat predicted by the Tanita, the Bodystat and skinfolds. Correlations between the resistance index (from the Tanita and Bodystat) with FFM were compared using the method described by Meng et al. [16] for comparing correlated correlations.

Correlational analysis shows if two measures are related to each other. However, it does not show if the two measures agree with each other. To assess the extent to which the: (a) impedance values measured from leg-to-leg (Tanita BIA system) agreed with the impedance values measured from arm-to-leg (Bodystat BIA system), and (b) percent fat predictions from the Tanita BIA (leg-to-leg) analysis system agreed with percent fat predictions from skinfolds, levels of agreement were calculated as described by Bland and Altman [17]. The consensus of opinion suggests that this is the most appropriate technique for the assessment of measurement agreement [18]. The average bias and 95% confidence interval for the bias was calculated for impedance and percent fat results for both genders separately. The differences between skinfold and Tanita predictions of percent fat were not normally distributed which affects the accuracy of the limits of agreement. Log transformation of the data, as recommended by Bland and Altman [17], resulted in a normal distribution of the differences between skinfold and Tanita predictions of percent fat. Alpha was set at 0.05 and, where stated, was adjusted to account for multiple comparisons.

Results

Impedance

Leg-to-leg impedance was significantly lower than arm-to-leg impedance ($F_{(1,32)} = 409.82$, $p < 0.001$; fig. 1). However, the two measures of impedance were highly correlated for both genders ($p < 0.001$; table 1). No main effect of gender or interaction of method × gender was found.

For each gender there were two correlations between stature-corrected impedance and FFM (table 2). To control for type 1 error the Bonferroni technique was used [19]. Alpha was divided by the number of tests being performed, $0.05/2 = 0.025$. Correlations were significant for both boys and girls for both the Tanita leg-to-leg BIA system and the Bodystat arm-to-leg BIA system. Correlations with FFM using the leg-to-leg resistance index (Tanita) were not significantly different to the arm-to-leg resistance index. Figure 1 shows that the impedance values measured by the Tanita leg-to-leg

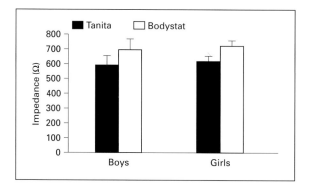

Fig. 1. Impedance by method and gender. Bodystat (arm-to-leg) impedance was significantly higher than Tanita (leg-to-leg) impedance (p<0.001).

Table 1. Correlations between impedance measurements

	Bodystat impedance	
	males	females
Tanita impedance	0.900	0.724

Males n = 17, females n = 17. All correlations significant p<0.001.

Table 2. Correlations between stature-corrected impedance values and fat free mass predicted from the equation of Slaughter et al. [13]

	Tanita stature-corrected impedance*		Bodystat stature-corrected impedance**	
	males	females	males	females
Fat-free mass, kg	0.965	0.841	0.972	0.873

Males n = 17, females n = 16. All correlations significant p<0.001.
* = (Height²)/(Tanita impedance); ** = (height²)/(Bodystat impedance).

system were consistently about 100 Ω lower than impedance measured by the Bodystat arm-to-leg system in both boys and girls (p<0.001; table 4).

For both boys and girls, the 95% limits showed that impedance scores from the Tanita BIA system were 51–164 Ω lower than impedance scores from the Bodystat BIA system (table 4).

Table 3. Correlations between skinfold, Tanita and Bodystat predictions of percent body fat

	Bodystat		Tanita	
	males	females	males	females
Skinfolds, % fat	0.810	0.869	0.733	0.926
Bodystat, % fat			0.714	0.955

Males n = 17, females n = 17. All correlations significant p < 0.005.

Percent Fat

As expected, girls had a higher mean percentage body fat than boys ($F_{(1,32)} = 21.10$, p < 0.001). Additionally, there was a significant main effect for prediction method ($F_{(2,64)} = 13.47$, p < 0.001) and a significant gender by prediction method interaction ($F_{(2,64)} = 7.86$, p = 0.001) on percent fat.

Follow-up Tukey's tests showed that in girls both the Tanita and Bodystat BIA systems predicted a higher mean percent body fat than skinfolds (p < 0.01), but not a significantly different mean percent fat from each other. In boys there were no differences between mean percent fat predicted by any of the methods.

For each gender there were 3 correlations between methods of assessing body fat. Alpha was adjusted as described above; 0.05/3 giving an alpha level of 0.017. All methods of predicting percent fat correlated significantly with each other (p < 0.005). This was true for boys and girls (table 3). Despite the significant differences between the mean percent fat predictions for girls (p < 0.01; fig. 2) the correlations were consistently lower for boys.

Levels of agreement showed that in about 95% of cases the percent fat scores predicted by the Tanita BIA could range from 37.6% below to 68.8% above the skinfold prediction of percent fat in boys, and from 3% below to 52% above the skinfold prediction of percent fat in girls (table 5). Note, because the data were logged before this analysis, the limits of agreement are not given in the units of their measurement (percent fat). Instead, the data can be interpreted as the percentage above or below the value for the skinfold prediction of percent fat.

Discussion

The accuracy of the prediction of children's FFM from stature-corrected impedance was the same irrespective of whether leg-to-leg impedance (Tanita)

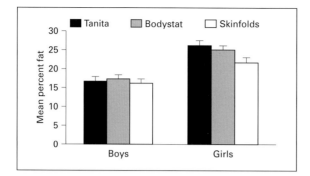

Fig. 2. Predicted percent fat by method and gender. For girls mean percent fat predicted by the Tanita and the Bodystat was higher than the mean percent fat predicted by skinfolds (p<0.01).

or arm-to-leg impedance (Bodystat) was used (table 2). This supports similar findings in adult subjects [8]. Additionally, there was no significant difference between percent fat predicted from leg-to-leg impedance and percent fat predicted from arm-to-leg impedance (fig. 1). However, in girls, but not boys, both BIA systems over estimated percent fat relative to percent fat predicted by skinfolds.

The correlations between stature-corrected impedance and FFM compare well with earlier research. In adults, Nunez et al. [8] found correlations of 0.93 and 0.89 (p<0.001) between FFM and arm-to-leg stature-corrected impedance and FFM and leg-to-leg stature-corrected impedance, respectively. These are slightly lower than the results from the current study for boys (arm-to-leg r=0.972, leg-to-leg r=0.965, both p<0.001) and slightly higher than the results for girls (arm-to-leg r=0.873, leg-to-leg r=0.841, both p<0.001). Eston et al. [9] also found higher correlations for boys than girls between FFM and arm-to-leg stature-corrected resistance (boys r=0.96, girls r=0.74, both p<0.001).

Previous studies have examined resistance and/or reactance components of impedance rather than impedance alone [9, 10]. The output from the leg-to-leg BIA unit used in this study does not provide these measures for comparison. However, an earlier study of 94 Caucasian 10- to 14-year-olds showed no difference in the accuracy of the prediction of FFM whether stature-corrected resistance (r=0.94, p<0.001), stature-corrected impedance (r=0.94, p<0.001) or stature-corrected resistance and reactance (r=0.95, p<0.001) were used [10]. This indicates that any of the above components can be used to predict FFM with equal accuracy.

Table 4. Levels of agreement for impedance measured by the Tanita BIA system and the Bodystat BIA system

	Impedance			
	BIAS (mean difference)	SD	95% limits ($\pm \Omega$)	95% limits of impedance scores from the Tanita BIA system relative to the Bodystat BIA system
Boys Tanita impedance and Bodystat impedance	–102.71	31.67	62.07	–164.77 to –40.64 Ω
Girls Tanita impedance and Bodystat impedance	–107.59	28.84	56.52	–164.10 to –51.07 Ω

Although correlated significantly (boys $r = 0.90$, girls $r = 0.72$, both $p < 0.001$), leg-to-leg impedance was about 100 Ω lower ($p < 0.001$) than arm-to-leg impedance (fig. 1; table 4). This is not surprising as body fat is not distributed evenly throughout the body. The legs would be expected to have a higher proportion of lean tissue than the trunk in both sexes, and hence be a better conductor. Due to this difference in impedance, it is important that equations developed for predicting FFM, percent fat or total body water (TBW) from arm-to-leg BIA are not used with impedance or resistance values obtained from the leg-to-leg system. At present the only available predictions for children's body composition using leg-to-leg BIA are the equations built into the Tanita system. Levels of body fat are a sensitive issue and these units are freely available in the shops, potentially to people with no understanding of the principles or limitations of BIA. Hence, it is important that the percent fat prediction is reasonably accurate.

The percent fat predicted from these equations in the Tanita system did not differ from those predicted by the Bodystat unit. However, in girls the percent fat was higher ($p < 0.01$) than percent fat predicted by skinfolds. This contrasts with the study by Eston et al. [9] who found that percent fat predicted by BIA was consistently lower than percent fat predicted by skinfolds. The skinfold equations used in Eston et al.'s [9] study to predict body fat were based on a multicomponent model, however, they were not the same equations as used in the present study. Eston et al. [9] stated that the predictive accuracy of the skinfold equations used resulted in systematic differences to original estimates when applied to published data. Additionally, the subjects were Chinese and aged 11–17 years, hence they were of a different pubertal and ethnic status to the present sample. Lohman [20] reported that FFM may be affected by ethnicity.

Table 5. Levels of agreement for log of percent fat predicted by skinfolds and Tanita BIA

		% fat		
		BIAS (log) (mean difference)	SD (log)	(antilog) 95% limits of % fat scores from Tanita impedance relative to skinfold prediction of % fat
Boys	log Tanita impedance and log skinfold prediction of % fat	1.13×10^{-2}	0.11	Tanita prediction = 37.6% below to 68.8% above skinfold prediction
Girls	log Tanita impedance and log skinfold prediction of % fat	8.46×10^{-2}	0.05	Tanita prediction = 3.0% below to 52.0% above skinfold prediction

Predictions of percent fat by the Tanita BIA system were significantly higher than skinfold predictions for girls, but not for boys. However, the 95% limits of agreement showed a bias to overestimation of percent fat in both genders, but particularly in girls (table 5). A boy measuring 15% body fat predicted by skinfolds may be predicted as anywhere between 9.4 and 25.3% by the Tanita BIA system. A girl measuring 25% body fat predicted by skinfolds may be predicted as anywhere between 24.3 and 38.0% by the Tanita BIA system (table 5). Thus, although the percentage over and under estimation may be smaller in girls, it is almost always an overestimation. Additionally, as girls typically carry more body fat than boys ($p < 0.001$), a smaller percentage overestimation may equate to the same or a larger actual overestimation. As girls are very susceptible to a fear of fatness [21] this overestimation has important implications.

Correlations between different methods of predicting percent fat were consistently higher for girls than boys (table 3), despite the significant differences in the predictions of percent fat for girls. This may be a function of the narrower range of scores in the boys' data, which would elicit lower correlations [22].

It is important to assess the levels of agreement of the Tanita against a recognised gold standard, for example, dual energy X-ray absorptiometry (DXA) or alternatively hydrodensitometry (with a multicomponent approach for the prediction of percent fat).

In summary, stature-corrected impedance using the leg-to-leg BIA system with pressure footpads explains as much variance in FFM as the traditional gel electrode arm-to-leg method. The prediction of percent fat provided by the system is not significantly different to that provided by the traditional arm-to-leg system. However, for girls both BIA predictions are significantly higher than predictions using skinfolds. For girls, the 95% limits of agreement show that the Tanita BIA system may overestimate or underestimate the skinfold prediction of percent fat by 52 and 3%, respectively. For boys, the 95% limits of agreement show that the Tanita BIA system may overestimate or underestimate the skinfold prediction of percent fat by 68.8 and 37.6%, respectively. Although the range is larger for boys the error for girls is almost consistently an overestimation. As the regression equation inside the Tanita is the only one available for children using leg-to-leg impedance analysis, and as this unit is marketed towards homes and health clubs, it is the accuracy of the unit as a whole, including the percent fat output, that is of current concern. The levels of agreement indicate that while average group values are reasonable, individual error may be unacceptable, particularly to people who are borderline obese or very thin.

However, this is an initial study on a relatively small sample. The system is extremely easy to use, provides a quick measurement and does not worry children or require the removal of any clothes other than shoes and socks. The high correlations of the stature-corrected impedance with FFM are very promising. Further research needs to use a gold standard criterion measure, such as the DXA, to assess the validity of the Tanita output, and to assess if there is a need to develop alternative regression equations. The day-to-day reliability of the Tanita BIA system also needs to be investigated.

References

1   Lean MEJ, Han TS, Seidell JC: Impairment of health and quality of life in people with large waist circumference. Lancet, 1998;351:853–856.
2   Charney E, Goodman HC, McBride M, Lyon B, Pratt R, Breese B, Disney F, Marx K: Childhood antecedents of adult obesity: Do chubby infants become obese adults? N Engl J Med 1976;295: 6–9.
3   Gutin B, Islam S, Manos T, Cucuzzo N, Smith C, Stachura M: The relations of percent fat and maximal aerobic capacity to risk factors for atherosclerosis and diabetes in black and white seven-to-eleven year old children. J Pediatr 1994;125:847–852.
4   Troiano RP, Flegal KM, Kuczmarski RJ, Campbell SM, Johnson CL: Overweight prevalence and trends for children and adolescents: The National Health and Nutrition Examination Surveys, 1963–1991. Arch Pediatr Adolesc Med 1995;149:1085–1091.
5   Kuczmarski RJ, Flegal KM, Campbell SM, Johnson CL: Increasing prevalence of overweight among US adults: The National Health and Nutrition Examination Surveys (NHANES), 1960–1991. JAMA 1994;272:205–211.
6   Ross JG, Pate RR, Lohman TG, Christenson GM: Changes in the body composition of children. The National Children and Youth Fitness Study II. JOPERD 1987:74–77.
7   Cerami R: Anesthetic conditions with anorexia nervosa. AANAJ 1993;61:165–169.
8   Nunez C, Gallagher D, Visser M, Pi-Sunyer FX, Wang Z, Heymsfield SB: Bioimpedance analysis: Evaluation of leg-to-leg system based on pressure contact footpad electrodes. Med Sci Sports Exerc 1997;29:524–531.
9   Eston RG, Cruz A, Fu F, Fung LM: Fat-free mass estimation by bioelectrical impedance and anthropometric techniques in Chinese children. J Sports Sci 1993;11:241–247.

10 Houtkooper LB, Lohman TG, Going SB, Hall MC: Validity of bioelectrical impedance for body composition assessment in children. J Appl Physiol 1989;66:814–821.

11 Goran MI, Kaskoun MC, Carpenter WH, Poehlman ET, Ravussin E, Fontvieille AM: Estimating body composition of young children by using bioelectrical resistance. J Appl Physiol 1993;75: 1776–1780.

12 Lohman TG: Applicability of body composition techniques and constants for children and youths; in Pandolph K (ed): Exercise and Sports Sciences Reviews. New York, Macmillan, 1986, pp 325–357.

13 Slaughter MH, Lohman TG, Boileau RA, Horswill CA, Stillman RJ, Van Loan MD, Bemben DA: Skinfold equations for estimation of body fatness in children and youth. Hum Biol 1988;60:709–723.

14 Janz KF, Nielsen DH, Cassady SL, Cook JS, Wu YT, Hansen JR: Cross-validation of the Slaughter skinfold equations for children and adolescents. Med Sci Sports Exerc 1993;25:1070–1076.

15 Graves JE, Pollock ML, Calvin AB, Van Loan M, Lohman TG: Comparison of different bioelectrical impedance analysers in the prediction of body composition. Am J Hum Biol 1989;1:603–611.

16 Meng XL, Rosenthal R, Rubin DB: Comparing correlated correlation coefficients. Psychol Bull 1992;111:172–175.

17 Bland JM, Altman DG: Statistical methods for assessing agreement between two methods of clinical measurement. Lancet 1986;i:307–310.

18 Nevill AM, Atkinson G: Assessing agreement between measurements recorded on a ratio scale in sports medicine and sports science. Br J Sports Med 1997;31:314–318.

19 Huck SW, Cormier WH: Reading Statistics and Research, ed 2. New York, Harper Collins, 1996, pp 312–313.

20 Lohman TG: Assessment of body composition in children. Pediatr Exerc Sci 1989;1:19–30.

21 Flynn MA: Fear of fatness and adolescent girls: Implications for obesity prevention. Proc Nutr Soc 1997;56:305–317.

22 Ferguson GA: Statistical Analysis in Psychology and Education, ed 5. New York, McGraw Hill, 1981, p 135.

Dr. Ann V. Rowlands, School of Sport, Health and Exercise Sciences,
University of Wales, Bangor LL57 2PX (UK)
Tel. +44 1248 383486, Fax +44 1248 371053, E-Mail a.rowlands@bangor.ac.uk

Jürimäe T, Hills AP (eds): Body Composition Assessment in Children and Adolescents.
Med Sport Sci. Basel, Karger, 2001, vol 44, pp 25–35

....

Measurement of Total Body Protein in Childhood

Louise A. Baur [a], *Jane R. Allen* [b], *Ian R. Humphries* [b], *Kevin J. Gaskin* [b]

[a] Department of Paediatrics and Child Health, University of Sydney, and
[b] James Fairfax Institute of Paediatric Clinical Nutrition, Royal Alexandra Hospital
for Children, Westmead, Sydney NSW, Australia

Total Body Protein

An accurate and precise measure of total body protein 'stores' in childhood would allow the relationship between body protein and growth, in both health and disease, to be explored. It would also permit the effect of different disease processes on total body protein to be better understood. However, one of the concerns with almost all of the indirect techniques used to assess lean mass or total body protein in childhood is that they are based on assumptions that may not be valid in situations of abnormal body composition, such as with wasting or fluid and electrolyte derangements [1, 2]. In addition, many of the body composition techniques have been inadequately evaluated, even in the normal paediatric population.

The measurement of total body nitrogen by neutron capture analysis offers the possibility of directly assessing body protein content. This technique is now well established for use in adult subjects [3–6]. How appropriate is it for use in childhood, and what information can be learnt from using it? A series of studies performed over several years at the Royal Alexandra Hospital for Children in Sydney has provided some answers to these questions [2, 7–15].

Measurement of Total Body Nitrogen

In the late 1970s and early 1980s, in vivo prompt gamma neutron activation analysis became well established as a technique for the measurement of the elemental composition of the human body. The basic principle of the technique is the detection of gamma-rays produced by interaction of a neutron (obtained from a neutron beam directed at the body) with the element of interest. There are two separate neutron activation techniques: the prompt-gamma technique and the delayed-gamma technique [16]. When a nucleus absorbs a neutron, the resultant compound nucleus is in an excited state. If there is subsequent emission of a gamma ray as part of the decay process of the excited nucleus (denoted n, γ), then this is termed 'radiative capture'. It is this process which is measured with the prompt-gamma technique. However, decay of the compound nucleus may occur by emission of nucleons (that is neutron, proton, alpha particle) followed by the production of one or more activation products. The gamma emission of these activation products can be measured, this process being termed the delayed-gamma technique. As a result of these two methods of neutron activation analysis, it is now possible to obtain absolute measurements of such elements as nitrogen, calcium, sodium, chlorine, phosphorous and carbon [16, 17].

The prompt-gamma method for measuring total body nitrogen (TBN), more properly termed 'prompt-gamma neutron capture analysis', was initially reported in the early 1970s [18]. The subject is exposed to a neutron source (e.g. ^{252}Cf or ^{238}Pu-Be); ^{14}N is converted to ^{15}N with the emission of a 10.8 MeV gamma ray which is specific for nitrogen [16]. By measuring TBN, total body protein can then be determined using the following relationship: mass of protein $= 6.25 \times$ mass of nitrogen. While several facilities for the measurement of TBN have been established, it essentially remains a research tool rather than a technique used for routine clinical measurement of body composition.

In the 1980s, a TBN facility was established in Sydney [5, 8] and a second TBN facility was established a decade later [13]. Two characteristics of the Sydney TBN facilities have made them particularly suitable for paediatric use. Firstly, they were designed as comparatively low-dose radiation facilities: a single TBN measurement gives a total body radiation dose $< \sim 0.25$ mSv (Quality Factor for neutrons $= 20$) in a 20-kg child [8, 13]. Secondly, the facilities are sufficiently accurate and precise for the measurement of small subjects, having an accuracy of 97–103% and a precision of 1.4–5.4% in the measurement of nitrogen mass in child-sized box and anthropomorphic phantoms [8, 13]. As a result of these features, it has been possible to perform direct measurement of TBN in normal children in a safe, accurate and reproducible manner.

The process of TBN measurement involves the subject resting on a table which moves the subject through a collimated beam of low-energy neutrons produced during the decay of ^{252}Cf. The resultant gamma-ray emission from the subject is measured by NaI (Tl) detectors placed on either side of the subject and perpendicular to both the neutron beam and the table direction. The total measurement time is less than 15 min [8].

Ethics approval for the studies summarised in this chapter was granted by the Human Ethics Committee of the Royal Alexandra Hospital for Children in Sydney.

Total Body Nitrogen Measurements in Normal Children

What is known of the body protein content of normal children? There have been a few early reports of body protein content in children based upon the chemical analysis of the carcasses of deceased children [19, 20]. Apart from these studies, body protein content has only been previously determined in children using *indirect* techniques. In the early 1980s, Fomon, Haschke and co-workers published the first detailed estimates of the body composition of the growing child and the adolescent male [21, 22]. Values for body protein at different ages were included, these estimates being based upon measurements of total body potassium.

The *direct* measurement of body protein content, by in vivo prompt-gamma neutron capture analysis, has the potential to produce very useful information. Firstly, the relationship between body protein and growth (not only of height and weight, but also of body compartment sizes) can be investigated, thereby providing insights into the normal physiology of growth in children. The acquisition of cross-sectional and longitudinal data can give more accurate information on protein accretion with age. Finally, it can provide control data, vital for the interpretation of TBN measurements in children with malnutrition due to a variety of causes.

We used the technique of in vivo prompt-gamma neutron capture analysis to determine the relationship between TBN and various growth indices in a group of 43 unselected normal children (18 males, 25 females) [9, 11, 14]. All were in good health and all had height and weight parameters that fell within two standard deviations of the normal population median for age (mean $\pm$ SD: -0.02 ± 0.92 and -0.06 ± 0.76 for height and weight SD scores, respectively). Ages ranged from 4.0 to 16.2 years (mean $\pm$ SD: 10.3 ± 3.3 years) at the time of study. Twenty-seven of the children were prepubertal and 16 (4 males, 12 females) were pubertal. There were no significant differences in anthropometric or body composition results for males and females in this particular study and so the data were pooled. A sex difference in these parameters, particularly in the older children, would have been expected and its absence may merely reflect the relatively small sample size for the study.

The relationship between TBN and age is displayed graphically in figure 1. With increasing age there is an increase in TBN, although, as expected, there is a wider spread of TBN values in the pubertal age group than in the younger

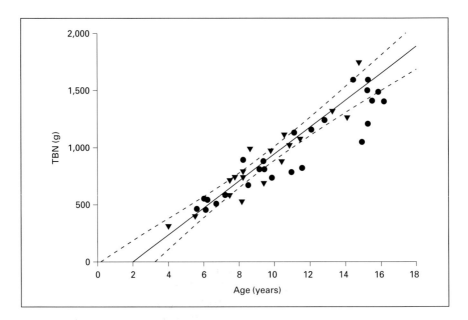

Fig. 1. TBN vs. age for 43 normal children. The regression line is shown with the dotted lines representing the 95% confidence intervals (see table 1). ▼ = Male; ● = female.

children. The equation for the line of best fit for this relationship is shown graphically in table 1, along with the regression equations for TBN versus height, weight or lean body mass (LBM; determined from skinfolds). There is a strong linear relationship between TBN and either height, weight or LBM for the children in this study. A similar relationship has also been shown between total body potassium (TBK) and the same anthropometric variables in normal children [23, 24]. This is not surprising, as both TBN and TBK closely reflect muscle mass, and growth of muscle mass would be associated with growth in height, weight and LBM.

The data in table 1 can also be used to provide preliminary information on the relationship, in normal children, between nitrogen deposition and the changes in anthropometric variables that occur during growth. The slope of the regression equation describing the relationship between TBN and age shows that, in general, 101 g nitrogen is gained per year of age over the age-range 4–16 years. Similarly, by considering the regression equations involving height or weight, it can be seen that approximately 19.9 g nitrogen is gained per cm of height gain and approximately 27.8 g nitrogen is gained per kg of weight gain. Estimated nitrogen deposition rates for just the prepubertal sub-group of children (n = 27) were similar: 96 g of nitrogen per year of age, 16.3 g

Table 1. TBN regression equations for 43 normal children*

Regression equation	r	95% CI	p
$TBN_N = -111 + 101 \times age_N$	0.93	0.87, 0.96	<0.001
$TBN_N = -1821 + 19.9 \times height_N$	0.96	0.93, 0.98	<0.001
$TBN_N = -34.0 + 27.8 \times weight_N$	0.97	0.94, 0.98	<0.001
$TBN_N = -295 + 46.0 \times LBM_N$	0.98	0.96, 0.99	<0.001

* Subscript $_N$ denotes normal group.
Units of measurement: TBN (g), age (years), height (cm), weight (kg), LBM (kg).
CI = Confidence intervals; LBM = lean body mass.

per cm of height gain and 26.7 g per kg of weight gain. These unique data have the potential to be used in estimating protein requirements in childhood. For instance, the current WHO guidelines for dietary protein intake [25] are based in part upon an estimate of the mean rate of nitrogen accretion during growth, values for which have been provided by the indirect estimates of Fomon et al. [21].

The above results for nitrogen deposition were obtained from cross-sectional studies. However, they have been supported by a study in which 17 healthy prepubertal children had two TBN measurements performed over a mean time period of 1.2 ± 0.6 years [14]. There was a wide range in nitrogen deposition recorded (–23 to 187 g per year), with a mean value of 77 g per year. This value is somewhat lower than that obtained using the cross-sectional data from the 43 children even when just the data for the prepubertal subgroup are considered.

The longitudinal study of 17 healthy prepubertal children has also provided information on the anthropometric associations with nitrogen deposition. The rate of nitrogen deposition was significantly and positively correlated with both weight velocity and the rate of deposition of LBM ($r_s = 0.49$, $p < 0.05$ and $r_s = 0.62$, $p = 0.01$, respectively), but there was no significant correlation with height velocity [14]. This finding at first appears counterintuitive as one would expect that changes in TBN would be accompanied by incremental changes in not only weight and LBM, but also height. Interestingly, a similar observation was made in a study of nitrogen deposition in a group of malnourished children with cystic fibrosis who were undergoing nutritional rehabilitation: nitrogen deposition was significantly correlated with weight gain but not height gain [9].

The cross-sectional data on TBN from the larger group of children can be used to give information about the timing of the development of chemical

Table 2. Relationship between age and TBN ratios for 43 normal children*

Regression equation	r	95% CI	p
$TBN_N/height_N = 1.39 + 0.50 \times age_N$	0.91	0.84, 0.95	<0.001
$TBN_N/weight_N = 23.4 + 0.31 \times age_N$	0.40	0.11, 0.63	<0.05
$TBN_N/LBM_N = 23.7 + 1.00 \times age_N$	0.77	0.63, 0.88	<0.001

* Subscript $_N$ denotes normal group.
Units of measurement: TBN (g), age (years), height (cm), weight (kg), LBM (kg).
CI = Confidence intervals; LBM = lean body mass.

maturity. Table 2 summarises the regression equations for the relationships between TBN and the ratios TBN/height, TBN/weight and TBN/LBM in these 43 children. There is a positive correlation between all three ratios and age (although weakest for TBN/weight). Thus, with increasing age, there is an increase in TBN per unit of height, weight or LBM in these normal children. In effect, children appear to become more 'nitrogen-concentrated' as they grow.

Moulton [26] defined chemical maturity as 'the point at which the concentration of water, proteins and salts becomes comparatively constant in the fat-free cell …'. He suggested that chemical maturity in humans was achieved at about the age of four years, the 'adult' nitrogen concentration being approximately 33 g/kg fat-free tissue. More recently, the theoretical calculations of Fomon et al. [21] and Haschke [22] have suggested that the nitrogen content of the fat-free mass gradually increases during childhood and adolescence, the value for an 18-year-old adolescent male being estimated at 32.5 g/kg. Our results show that the nitrogen content of LBM is significantly age-dependent over the range of ages studied (4–16 years). In addition, the mid-teenage TBN/height ratio of 8–11 g/cm is in close agreement with published values for adult subjects [3, 27]. These results therefore provide strong evidence that chemical maturity, at least for nitrogen content, does not occur until the mid-teen years. It is probable that this is related to the timing of puberty and hence may also be sex dependent. A larger sample size would be needed to explore this more fully.

How do our data compare with results from previous studies? The data for prepubertal children are in reasonable agreement with the only previous estimates of TBN in normal children [21]. However, the current data should be regarded as the more authoritative, especially with respect to the relationships between TBN and height, weight and age, in that they represent, uniquely, direct measurements, in contrast with the TBK-derived estimates of TBN in the study of Fomon et al. [21].

Total Body Nitrogen in Children with Chronic Disease

Many chronic diseases in childhood are complicated by the development of short stature. Depending upon the disease, various factors may contribute to this growth failure including energy deficient diets, an elevation in energy expenditure, fluid and electrolyte disorders and various endocrine and genetic abnormalities [28]. In normal children, linear growth is dependent upon an adequate nutrient intake and subsequent nitrogen accretion or protein deposition [21]. What happens to nitrogen accretion in children with chronic disease? Is there any pattern in its association with growth or short stature?

In order to answer these questions we performed TBN measurements in seven different 'disease' groups of children [9, 10, 12, 14, 15], as follows:

(i) 16 prepubertal males with idiopathic short stature (height SD-score <-2.00);

(ii) 17 children (10 male; 9 prepubertal) with chronic renal failure and short stature (height SD-score <-2.00) [12].

(iii) 10 children (4 male; 9 prepubertal) with chronic liver disease who were awaiting liver transplantation;

(iv) 21 malnourished children (12 male; 12 prepubertal) with cystic fibrosis (CF) who were involved in a nutritional supplementation program [9];

(v) 31 children (10 male; 20 prepubertal) with juvenile chronic arthritis;

(vi) 37 prepubertal children (21 male) with phenylketonuria (PKU) [14];

(vii) 75 normally nourished children (41 male) with CF [15].

As can be seen from table 3, these children generally had mean values for height and weight SD-scores that were significantly below the population median value of zero, with the exception of the normally nourished CF children. In particular, the children with idiopathic short stature and chronic renal failure had greatly reduced height and weight SD-scores.

Table 3 also shows the TBN results for the different groups of children, expressed as a percentage of that predicted for age or height using equations derived from the data for the normal children as discussed previously. Apart from the normally nourished CF females, all groups had significantly reduced TBN values predicted for age. This finding was especially marked in the children with chronic renal failure, with the idiopathic short stature and malnourished CF groups being the next most severely depleted. Interestingly, when the TBN data were expressed as a percentage of that predicted for height, the renal failure, short stature, normally nourished CF and PKU groups

Table 3. Anthropometric and TBN data for the seven 'disease' groups (means ± SD)

Group	Age years	Height SD-score	Weight SD-score	TBN (age)[1]	TBN (height)[1]
Short stature	10.3 ± 3.3	–2.7 ± 0.4*	–1.8 ± 0.5*	69.8 ± 9.9[+]	99.3 ± 13.4
Renal failure	12.9 ± 3.2	–4.1 ± 1.4*	–2.4 ± 1.0*	54.2 ± 15.0[+]	100.2 ± 30.3
Liver disease	9.9 ± 4.2	–1.2 ± 1.5*	–0.1 ± 1.5	83.2 ± 27.7[+]	88.3 ± 19.5[+]
Malnourished CF	12.3 ± 3.1	–1.8 ± 0.9*	–1.8 ± 0.8*	70.2 ± 11.7[+]	85.5 ± 12.1[+]
Arthritis	10.0 ± 3.2	–0.7 ± 1.3*	–0.6 ± 1.3*	83.3 ± 23.6[+]	90.0 ± 21.1[+]
PKU	7.3 ± 2.0	–0.4 ± 0.9*	–0.1 ± 0.8	91.8 ± 14.8[+]	101.7 ± 16.3
Normally nourished					
CF males	10.6 ± 2.6	–0.3 ± 1.3	–0.2 ± 1.1	88.8 ± 23.0[+]	98.7 ± 13.5
CF females	10.2 ± 3.1	–0.1 ± 1.1	–0.1 ± 1.1	93.6 ± 16.2	101.4 ± 10.0

[1] TBN as a percentage of that predicted for age or height.
* Significantly different from 0 (population median) by t test, $p < 0.05$.
[+] Significantly different from 100% by t test, $p < 0.05$.
PKU = Phenylketonuria; CF = cystic fibrosis.

demonstrated values that were not significantly different from 100%. These groups thus had appropriate levels of TBN for height. The other three groups of patients (i.e. those with liver disease, malnourished CF or chronic arthritis) had mean levels of TBN predicted from height that were still reduced, although not as severely as when predicted from age.

Thus, the children in these different studies were all found to be severely nitrogen-depleted for age, with the exception of the normally nourished CF females. Presumably, therefore, the different conditions all resulted in chronic protein depletion and thus inadequate nitrogen accretion.

In four of the groups (namely short stature, renal failure, normally nourished CF males and PKU), nitrogen content was found to be appropriate for height but depleted for age. Two of these groups had marked short stature and all had little or no evidence of acute wasting. The exact mechanisms for the reduction in nitrogen accretion in these groups are not fully understood. Familial and constitutional factors may contribute to the reduced height growth in the idiopathic short stature group. Patients with chronic renal failure have been shown to consume energy deficient diets [29] and this may be one of the factors promoting a poor rate of nitrogen deposition in these patients. In the PKU patients, the restriction of phenylalanine at an earlier age may have played a role in limiting nitrogen accretion. Whatever the cause, the resultant long-term decrease in nitrogen gain appears to have led to a proportionate decrease in height gain. In these patients, body protein is thus appropriate for height, whilst being depleted for age.

In the remaining three groups of children (that is, malnourished CF, chronic liver disease and chronic arthritis) the mean values for TBN as a percentage of that predicted for height were significantly reduced. This finding may be due to the fact that all three groups included individuals with acute wasting (decreased weight for height) complicating their chronic disease. A relatively acute nutritional insult could lead to decreased nitrogen accretion and weight loss with, of course, no effect on height in the short term. The result would be a reduction in body protein adjusted for either height or age. Note that in these three groups of children, this acute process could be superimposed on the process of chronic protein depletion.

A possible interpretation of these findings is that acute protein depletion in the growing child may be associated with nitrogen depletion for both age and height. However, long-term inadequacy of protein deposition, from whatever cause, will result in a reduced body protein content for age, an appropriate body nitrogen content for height and stunting of height. This suggests that the degree of wasting of lean tissue (that is, acute protein energy malnutrition) may be able to be quantified by the degree of deviation below the TBN predicted for height.

Conclusions

In a series of studies performed over several years in Sydney, we have demonstrated that TBN can be measured safely and adequately in children by the technique of in vivo prompt-gamma neutron capture analysis. Using this technique it has been possible to describe the relationships between body protein content and growth indices in the healthy growing child. TBN measurement has also allowed us to quantify the degree of protein depletion caused by a chronic disease process in a child, as well as show the close relationship between height and chronic protein depletion in the growing child. Finally, measurement of TBN has permitted acute and chronic protein malnutrition to be described, for the first time, in terms of changes in body protein content.

References

1   Lohman TG: Applicability of body composition techniques and constants for children and youths. Exerc Sport Sci Rev 1986;14:325–357.
2   Baur LA: Body composition in normal children – Ethical and methodological limitations. Asia Pac J Clin Nutr 1994;4:35–38.

3   Cohn SH, Vartsky D, Yasumura S, Sawitsky A, Zanzi I, Vaswani A, Ellis K: Compartmental body composition based on total-body nitrogen, potassium, and calcium. Am J Physiol 1980;239: E524–E530.

4   Beddoe AH, Zuidmeer H, Hill GL: A prompt gamma in vivo neutron activation analysis facility for measurement of total body nitrogen in the critically ill. Phys Med Biol 1984;29:371–383.

5   Allen BJ, Blagojevic N, McGregor BH, Parsons DE, Gaskin KJ, Soutter VL, Waters D, Allman M, Stewart P, Tiller D: In vivo determination of protein in malnourished patients; in Ellis KJ, Yasumura S, Morgan WD (eds): In vivo Body Composition Studies. London, Institute of Physical Sciences in Medicine, 1987, pp 77–82.

6   Ryde SJS, Morgan WD, Evans CJ, Sivyer A, Dutton J: Calibration and evaluation of a ^{252}Cf-based neutron activation analysis instrument for the determination of nitrogen in vivo. Phys Med Biol 1989;34:1429–1441.

7   Gaskin KJ, Waters DLM, Soutter VL, Baur LA, Soutter VL, Gruca MA: Nutritional status, growth and development in children undergoing intensive treatment for cystic fibrosis. Acta Paediatr Scand 1990;366(suppl):106–110.

8   Baur LA, Allen BJ, Rose A, Blagojevic N, Gaskin KJ: A total body nitrogen facility for paediatric use. Phys Med Biol 1991;36:1363–1375.

9   Baur LA, Waters DL, Allen BJ, Blagojevic N, Gaskin KJ: Nitrogen deposition in malnourished children with cystic fibrosis. Am J Clin Nutr 1991;53:503–511.

10   Baur LA, Allen BJ, Allen R, Cowell CT, Dorney SFA, Knight JF, Gaskin KJ: Total body nitrogen in idiopathic short stature and chronic diseases of childhood; in Ellis KJ, Eastman JD (eds): Human Body Composition. New York, Plenum Press, 1993, pp 143–146.

11   Baur LA, Allen JR, Waters DL, Gaskin KJ: Total body nitrogen in prepubertal children; in Ellis KJ, Eastman JD (eds): Human Body Composition. New York, Plenum Press, 1993, pp 139–142.

12   Baur LA, Knight JF, Crawford BA, Reed E, Roy LP, Gaskin KJ: Total body protein in children with chronic renal failure and short stature. Eur J Clin Nutr 1994;48:433–441.

13   Humphries IRJ, Allen BJ, Blagojevic N, Gaskin KJ: Hydrogen background in total body nitrogen estimations. Phys Med Biol 1995;40:201–207.

14   Allen JR, Baur LA, Waters DL, Allen BJ, Gaskin KJ: Body protein in prepubertal children with phenylketonuria. Eur J Clin Nutr 1996;50:178–186.

15   Allen JR, Humphries IRJ, McCauley JC, Waters DL, Allen BJ, Baur LA, Roberts DCK, Gaskin KJ: Assessment of body composition of children with cystic fibrosis. Appl Radiat Isot 1998;49: 591–592.

16   Chettle DR, Fremlin JH: Techniques of in vivo neutron activation analysis. Phys Med Biol 1984; 29:1011–1043.

17   Ryde SJS, Morgan WD, Sivyer A, Evans CJ, Dutton J: A clinical instrument for multi-element in vivo analysis by prompt, delayed and cyclic neutron activation using ^{252}Cf. Phys Med Biol 1987;32: 1257–1271.

18   Biggin HC, Chen NS, Ettinger KV, Fremlin JH, Morgan WD, Nowotny R: Determination of nitrogen in living patients. Nat New Biol 1972;36:187–188.

19   Widdowson EM, Dickerson JWT: Chemical composition of the body; in Comar CL, Bronner F (eds): Mineral Metabolism: An Advanced Treatise, vol II, part A. The Elements. New York, Academic Press, 1964, pp 2–247.

20   Garrow JS, Fletcher K, Halliday D: Body composition in severe infantile malnutrition. J Clin Invest 1965;44:417–425.

21   Fomon SJ, Haschke F, Ziegler EE, Nelson SE: Body composition of reference children from birth to age 10 years. Am J Clin Nutr 1982;35:1169–1175.

22   Haschke F: Body composition of adolescent males. I. Total body water in normal adolescent males. II. Body composition of the male reference adolescent. Acta Paediatr Scand 1983;307(suppl):1–23.

23   Flynn MA, Woodruff C, Clark J, Chase G: Total body potassium in normal children. Pediatr Res 1972;6:239–245.

24   Forbes GB, Hursh JB: Age and sex trends in lean body mass calculated from K^{40} measurements: With a note on the theoretical basis for the procedure. Ann NY Acad Sci 1963;110:255–263.

25   FAO/WHO/UNU: Energy and protein requirements. WHO Tech Rep Ser 724. Geneva, WHO, 1985.

26 Moulton CR: Age and chemical development in mammals. J Biol Chem 1923;57:79–97.

27 Cleland JGF, Dargie HJ, Robertson I, Robertson JIS, East BW: Total body electrolyte composition in patients with heart failure: A comparison with normal subjects and patients with untreated hypertension. Br Heart J 1987;58:230–238.

28 Underwood LE: Growth retardation in chronic diseases: Possible mechanisms. Acta Paediatr Suppl 1999;428:93–96.

29 Simmons JM, Wilson CJ, Potter DE, Holliday MA: Relation of calorie deficiency to growth failure in children on hemodialysis and the growth response to calorie supplementation. N Engl J Med 1971;285:653–656.

Assoc. Prof. Louise A. Baur, University of Sydney, Royal Alexandra Hospital for Children,
PO Box 3515, Parramatta NSW 2124 (Australia)
Tel. +61 2 9845 0000 (switchboard); +61 2 9845 3393 (direct), Fax +61 2 9845 3389
E-Mail louiseb3@nch.edu.au

Jürimäe T, Hills AP (eds): Body Composition Assessment in Children and Adolescents.
Med Sport Sci. Basel, Karger, 2001, vol 44, pp 36–45

....

The Relationship of Subcutaneous Adipose Tissue Topography (SAT-Top) by Means of LIPOMETER with Body Mass Index and Body Composition in Obese Children and Adolescents

Karl Sudi[a], *Reinhard Möller*[b], *Erwin Tafeit*[b], *Gudrun Weinhandl*[c],
Martin Helmuth Borkenstein[c]

[a] Institute for Sport Sciences;
[b] Institute for Medical Chemistry and Pregl Laboratory, and
[c] Division for Diabetes and Endocrinology, Pediatric Hospital, Karl-Franzens University,
Graz, Austria

Obesity in childhood is a public health problem in developed countries [1]. The criteria used to assess overweight and obesity vary widely and there is a need to define obesity in an appropriate manner, especially in the pediatric population [2].

The clinical assessment of body fat mass needs to be quick, cheap, repeatable, safe and noninvasive [3]. Anthropometric characteristics, e.g. body mass index (BMI) [4] and available standard methods, such as bioelectrical impedance (BIA) are widely used in field studies and in the clinical setting although hydration of fat free mass [5] and regional adiposity might influence the prediction of impedance-derived fatness [6]. More advanced techniques such as computed tomography (CT), magnetic resonance imaging (MRI), or dual-energy X-ray absorptiometry are not available everywhere and are also limited in their application, either due to high costs (MRI) or radiological burden (CT).

We have shown recently that an optical device, LIPOMETER, allows the determination of subcutaneous adipose tissue thickness at arbitrarily chosen body sites in a rapid, safe, and noninvasive manner [7, 8]. Fifteen well-defined body sites were specified to standardize measurements providing an estimate of subcutaneous adipose topography (SAT Top) of the human body [9]. As both body composition and body fat distribution changes with adiposity and

Table 1. Anthropometric characteristics and values of summed SAT layers in obese boys and girls

Parameters	Boys (n = 84)	Girls (n = 124)	p (ANOVA)
Age, years	11.8 ± 2.1 [4.4–17.5]	11.9 ± 1.8 [7.9–16.4]	0.62
Body mass, kg	66.1 ± 17.45 [31–125]	67.2 ± 16.7 [36.7–113.2]	0.64
Height, cm	156.1 ± 12.3 [113–178.6]	155.9 ± 9.2 [135.5–177.1]	0.85*
BMI	26.7 ± 3.9 [19.65–44.5]	27.3 ± 4.8 [19–42.1]	0.48*
Fat mass, kg	29.2 ± 10.3 [9.9–72]	31.6 ± 11.7 [11.9–65.25]	0.13
% fat mass	43.85 ± 6.5 [23.5–57.6]	45.9 ± 7.1 [25.7–61]	0.037
Σ1–6, mm	93.3 ± 25.6 [38.8–187.2]	98.3 ± 28.8 [30.2–164.7]	0.205
Σ7–10, mm	76.1 ± 18.1 [44.7–117.1]	74.6 ± 18.5 [33.8–124.9]	0.55
Σ11–15, mm	51 ± 12.8 [26.8–92]	46.5 ± 10.2 [22.1–75.7]	0.013*
Σ1–15, mm	220.4 ± 48 [125.5–378.7]	219.3 ± 45.8 [97.7–338]	0.87
Σ1–6/Σ7–10	1.24 ± 0.28 [0.63–2.17]	1.34 ± 0.38 [0.79–2.73]	0.12*
Σ1–6/Σ11–15	1.9 ± 0.61 [0.9–4.95]	2.2 ± 0.81 [0.9–5.2]	0.0065*

* By means of Kruskal-Wallis.

Data are shown as mean ± SD, and [range]. Abbreviations used: Σ1–6 = Sum of SAT layers from 1-neck to 6-lateral chest; Σ7–10 = sum of SAT layers from 7-upper abdomen to 10-hip; Σ11–15 = sum of SAT layers from 11-front thigh to 15-calf; Σ1–15 = sum of SAT layers from 1-neck to 15-calf; Σ1–6/Σ7–10 = ratio of upper body subcutaneous fat vs. trunk subcutaneous fat; Σ1–6/Σ11–15 = ratio of upper body subcutaneous fat vs. lower extremities subcutaneous fat.

age of children [10], we measured SAT Top in obese boys and girls and compared the relationship of measured SAT layers with estimates of adiposity, namely BMI and impedance-derived fatness.

Subjects and Methods

Subjects

84 obese boys (mean ± SD: age 11.8 ± 2.1 years, BMI (kg/m²) 26.7 ± 3.9) and 124 obese girls (age: 11.9 ± 1.8 years, BMI: 27.3 ± 4.8) were investigated. Obesity was defined as a BMI ≥ 90th percentile for age and sex. Anthropometric characteristics are shown in table 1.

Assessment of Body Composition

Fat free mass (FFM) of children was estimated by means of bioelectrical impedance (BIA Akern-RJL 101/S) with an applied current of 0.8 mA at 50 kHz in the fasting state after children were resting in supine position. The equation used to predict FFM has been established for the pediatric age range [3.9–19.3 years] by validating FFM predicted by BIA against potassium-dilution technique [11].

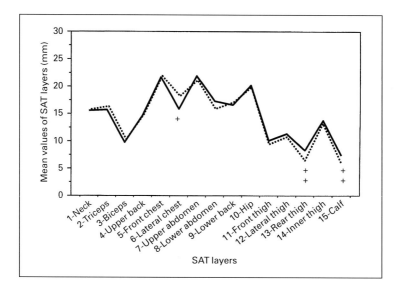

Fig. 1. Mean values of 15 measured SAT layers (from 1-neck to 15-calf) in boys (solid line) and girls (dotted line). Value of SAT layer 6-lateral chest was greater in girls, values of SAT layers 13-rear thigh and 15-calf were greater in boys, respectively. $^+$ p $<$ 0.01; $^{++}$ p $<$ 0.0001.

Fat mass (FM) was calculated as the difference between body mass and FFM. Percentage fat mass (% FM) was expressed as the relative amount of FM for a given body mass (table 1).

Assessment of Subcutaneous Adipose Tissue Layers (SAT Layers)

The thickness of SAT layers were measured by means of the optical device LIPOMETER (EU Patent No. 0516251). Briefly, the sensor head of the Lipometer consists of a set of light emitting diodes (LED) ($\lambda = 660$ nm, light intensity 3,000 mcd) as light sources and a photodetector. The LEDs illuminate the selected SAT layer, forming geometrical patterns that vary in succession. The photodiode measures the corresponding light intensities that are back-scattered in the SAT. These light signals are amplified, digitized and stored in a computer. Calibration and evaluation were done using CT as the reference [7].

Measurement for the thickness of SAT layers in mm are performed at 15 specified body sites, from 1-neck to 15-calf, on the right side of the body in a standing position (fig. 1). The coefficients of variation of SAT layers range between 1.9% for SAT layer 5-front chest and 12.2% for SAT layer 13-rear thigh [9].

Statistics

Kolmogorov-Smirnov test was used to prove normality of data. Data not normally distributed were normalised by means of Box-Cox Transformation. Analysis of variance (using the Bonferroni correction) was used to compare parameters between boys and girls. Kruskal-Wallis test was used if variances were not normally distributed. Correlations between variables of interest were calculated using Pearsons correlation coefficient and partial correlation was performed to adjust for the influence of confounding variables. Factor analysis for measured SAT layers (not shown) was employed to reduce the complex information of the data space and to reduce an unwarranted large number of correlations. The independence and significance of variables to contribute to the variation in relative fatness was tested by stepwise multiple regression analysis. The significance level of p values was set at 5%. Values of SAT layers are shown as mean scores (fig. 1), and all other values are given as mean, standard deviation, and range (table 1).

Results

In girls, SAT layers 3-biceps (p=0.028) and 9-lower back (p=0.044) were slightly skewed to the left. The thickness of SAT layer 6-lateral chest was greater in girls (18.4±7 mm) than in boys (15.9±5.65 mm; p=0.008). The thickness of SAT layers 13-rear thigh (boys: 8.3±3.3 mm; girls: 6.5±2 mm; p<0.0001) and 15-calf (boys: 7.4±2.25 mm; girls: 6.1±1.7 mm; p<0.0001) were greater in boys, respectively (fig. 1). Boys had a lower % FM than girls (p<0.04; table 1).

Factor analysis revealed that the information of measured SAT layers can be condensed by three factors which were the same for boys and for girls (not shown).

Factor 1 includes SAT layers from 1-neck to 6-lateral chest, factor 2 includes SAT layers from 11-front thigh to 15-calf, and factor 3 includes SAT layers from 7-upper abdomen to 10-hip. To provide a simple way to calculate values according to each of the factors extracted by factor analysis, a linear addition was performed for factor 1-related SAT layers (Σ1–6), factor 2-related SAT layers (Σ11–15) and factor 3-related SAT layers (Σ7–10) (table 1). To give a crude estimate of total subcutaneous fat, the sum of 15 SAT layers (Σ1–15) was also estimated (table 1). Additionally, two ratios were calculated. The first ratio of ΣSAT layers 1–6 and ΣSAT layers 7–10 (Σ1–6/Σ7–10) serves as an index of upper body subcutaneous fat distribution. The second ratio of ΣSAT layers 1–6 and ΣSAT layers 11–15 (Σ1–6/Σ11–15) serves as an index of upper body versus lower extremities subcutaneous fat distribution.

The sum of SAT layers from the lower extremities (Σ11–15) was greater in boys (p=0.013) whereas the ratio Σ1–6/Σ11–15 was higher in girls (p=0.0065; table 1).

Pearson Correlation

Anthropometric and body composition data were intercorrelated (table 2). Body mass and BMI (fig. 2) showed the highest correlation to FM. Body mass, FM, BMI (fig. 2), but not age were in relationship with % FM. The magnitude of these associations remained almost unchanged after adjustment for gender.

Table 2. Correlation between anthropometric characteristics, body composition data, sums and ratios of measured SAT layers

Parameters	Age	Body mass	BMI	FM	% FM
All children (n = 208)					
Age	–	0.66[++]	0.39[++]	0.49[++]	0.09
Body Mass	0.66[++]	–	0.88[++]	0.94[++]	0.59[++]
BMI	0.39[++]	0.88[++]	–	0.94[++]	0.75[++]
FM	0.49[++]	0.94[++]	0.94[++]	–	0.81[++]
% FM	0.09	0.59[++]	0.75	0.81	–
Boys (n = 84)					
Σ1–6	0.07	0.29[+]	0.385[++]	0.40	0.54[++]
Σ7–10	−0.31[+]	−0.21*	−0.09	−0.0	0.31[+]
Σ11–15	−0.18	−0.22*	−0.06	−0.0	0.315[+]
Σ1–15	−0.13	0.02	0.15	0.19*	0.48[++]
Σ1–6/Σ7–10	0.38[+]	0.61[++]	0.60[++]	0.57[++]	0.37[+]
Σ1–6/Σ11–15	0.25*	0.50[++]	0.42[++]	0.415[++]	0.25*
Girls (n = 124)					
Σ1–6	0.05	0.55[++]	0.68[++]	0.67[++]	0.75[++]
Σ7–10	−0.25[+]	−0.05	0.07	0.05	0.23[+]
Σ11–15	−0.16*	−0.29[+]	−0.21[+]	−0.25[+]	−0.12
Σ1–15	−0.1	0.26[+]	0.41[++]	0.39[++]	0.54[++]
Σ1–6/Σ7–10	0.30[+]	0.67[++]	0.70[++]	0.72[++]	0.64[++]
Σ1–6/Σ11–15	0.16*	0.66[++]	0.72[++]	0.72[++]	0.68[++]

*p < 0.05, [+]p < 0.01, [++]p < 0.0001.

In general, all different sums of SAT layers were associated with relative fatness (%FM) in boys, but not in girls. In girls, Σ11–15 was not significantly associated with %FM but was in significant inverse relationship with age, body mass, BMI, and FM (table 2). In boys, the relationship of overall subcutaneous fat, as reflected by Σ1–15 with BMI and FM was only of minor magnitude when compared with girls. Both calculated ratios were significantly associated with absolute and relative fatness in boys and in girls. Nevertheless, in boys Σ1–6/Σ7–10 was slightly higher associated with absolute and relative fatness than Σ1–6/Σ11–15 (fig. 4). In girls, the magnitude in the relationship of both ratios with absolute and relative fatness was nearly identical (fig. 4). However, in boys and in girls, Σ1–6 was the best associate of relative fatness (fig. 3).

We also performed partial correlation to adjust for the possible influence of chronologic age. In boys and in girls, the magnitude in the relationship of relative fatness with the different sums of SAT layers and with both calculated

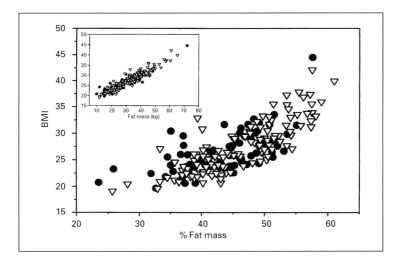

Fig. 2. Scatterplot shows the association between relative fatness (% FM) and BMI in obese boys (filled circles) and obese girls (open triangles). The small figure in the left corner (top) shows the association between absolute fatness (FM) and BMI.

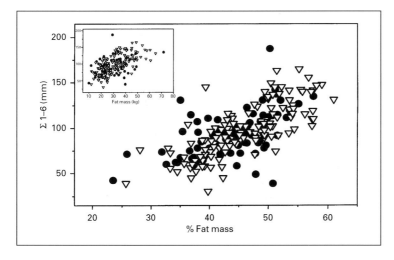

Fig. 3. Scatterplot shows the association between relative fatness (% FM) and upper body subcutaneous fat (Σ1–6) in obese boys (filled circles) and obese girls (open triangles). The small figure in the left corner (top) shows the association between absolute fatness (FM) and Σ1–6.

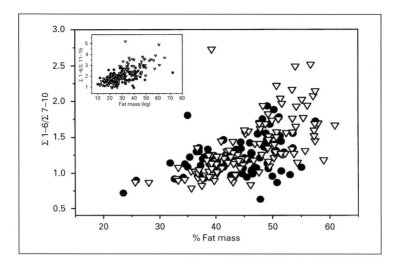

Fig. 4. Scatterplot shows the association between relative fatness (% FM) and the ratio of upper body subcutaneous fat vs. trunk subcutaneous fat ($\Sigma1$–$6/\Sigma7$–10) in obese boys (filled circles) and obese girls (open triangles). The small figure in the left corner (top) shows the association between absolute fatness (FM) and the ratio of upper body subcutaneous fat vs. lower extremities subcutaneous fat ($\Sigma1$–$6/\Sigma11$–15).

ratios, did not significantly change when adjusted for age. However, the association of absolute fatness with the different sums of SAT layers and calculated ratios seemed to be under a somewhat higher influence of chronologic age in boys when compared with girls perhaps due to the effects of unmeasured visceral fat in boys (not shown).

Multiple Regression Analysis

A stepwise model with relative fatness (% FM) as dependent variable was calculated for boys and girls separately. In boys, BMI (39.4%, $p < 0.0001$) together with $\Sigma1$–15 ($+15.5\%$, $p < 0.0001$) and age ($+1.7\%$, $p = 0.044$) explained 56.7% of the variation in % FM (adj. $R^2 = 0.567$, $p < 0.0001$). In girls, BMI (65.6%, $p < 0.0001$) together with $\Sigma1$–6 ($+7.4\%$, $p < 0.0001$) and age ($+1.7\%$, $p = 0.0033$) explained 74.7% of the variation in % FM (adj. $R^2 = 0.747$, $p < 0.0001$). In boys and in girls, age had a negative slope in the regression model.

Discussion

The thickness of 15 different SAT layers was measured in obese children with a similar pattern of SAT layers found in boys and girls (fig. 1). However, children in the present study were from 5 to 17 years of age and this range covers all stages of pubertal development. Because stages of maturation were not available, we cannot rule out the possibility that the pattern of SAT layers is different between, and within gender with respect to the stage of biological maturation [12].

Based on factor analysis, the sum of three subcutaneous fat compartments were calculated and correlated against body composition data. In boys, the sum of all three compartments was significantly associated with relative fatness. In girls, lower body subcutaneous fat for example $\Sigma 11-15$ was not associated with relative fatness (% FM) and was negatively related to BMI and fat mass (FM), even after controlling for age. Because lower body subcutaneous fat was negatively related to age in girls but not in boys, it is likely that subcutaneous fat increases predominantly on the upper aspect of the trunk with aging and accretion of FM, especially in obese girls. This, in part, can also be shown by the ratio of subcutaneous fat from the upper body versus that from the trunk, e.g. $\Sigma 1-6/\Sigma 7-10$ which is associated with all indices of fatness in both sexes, but predominantly in girls (table 2; fig. 4). Nevertheless, the evolution of this ratio also implies that an increase in body mass and FM in boys is associated with a relative decrease in subcutaneous fat from the trunk, e.g. $\Sigma 7-10$, and an increase in subcutaneous fat from the upper body, e.g. $\Sigma 1-6$. In girls, however, the decrease in subcutaneous fat from the lower extremities with ageing and increase in adiposity, is associated with a slight increase in the relationship of the ratio $\Sigma 1-6/\Sigma 11-15$ with fatness when compared with $\Sigma 1-6/\Sigma 7-10$ (table 2; fig. 4). Nevertheless, in both sexes independent of age, subcutaneous fat from the upper body, as reflected by $\Sigma 1-6$ showed the best association with relative fatness (% FM).

FM was calculated indirectly by means of impedance. The high correlation between FM, body mass, and BMI (fig. 2) may have its origin in the equation used. Besides impedance, age and height are the main components of the regression equation which predicts fat free mass [11]. Because age, body mass, and height are also strongly intercorrelated, this may have resulted in the obtained high correlations. Alternatively, it is also possible that the distribution of body fat in the upper body versus lower body has an impact on impedance, as shown previously in women [6]. Besides methodological concerns using bioelectrical impedance to estimate body composition, the results suggest that BMI can be used instead of FM to calculate absolute fatness in a homogenous group of obese children.

BMI and age contributed significantly to the variation in relative fatness in boys and in girls. However, the p value for the variable age was poor in boys, and age also had a negative slope in the regression model in boys and girls. Whereas in boys total subcutaneous fat, as reflected by $\Sigma 1-15$ contributed significantly to the variance, subcutaneous fat from the upper body, e.g. $\Sigma1$–6, was a significant component of the regression model in girls. Thus, gender-specific differences in the enlargement and distribution of subcutaneous fat depots should be considered when estimating relative fatness. Furthermore, the regression model explained a greater percentage of the variation in relative fatness in girls. The power of anthropometric characteristics, e.g. BMI and SAT layers, to predict relative fatness is therefore of greater magnitude in girls. Whether this could have its underlying reason in gender-dependent differences in growth spurts and/or in the amount of visceral fat, remains to be elucidated.

Conclusion and Perspectives

The study describes the associations between the sum and ratios of different SAT layers, anthropometric characteristics, and body composition in obese children. It may be concluded that the assessment of SAT layers and their distribution gives additional information for the estimation of fatness. There is great demand for methods which are safe, easy-to-handle, and repeatable to assess overall and regional adiposity. This novel device fulfils these criteria and could also be of help to define cut-off values to differentiate between overweight and obese and to monitor changes in the distribution of subcutaneous fat under several conditions.

References

1   Lehingue Y: The European Childhood Obesity Group (ECOG) project: the European collaborative study on the prevalence of obesity in children. Am J Clin Nutr 1999;70(suppl):166S–168S.
2   Guillaume M: Defining obesity in childhood: Current practice. Am J Clin Nutr 1999;70(suppl): 126S–130S.
3   Poskitt EME: Assessment of body composition in the obese; in Davies PSW, Cole TJ (eds): Body Composition Techniques in Health and Disease. Society for the Study of Human Biology Symposium, Series 36. Cambridge, University Press, 1995, pp 146–165.
4   Malina RM, Katzmarzyk PT: Validity of the body mass index as an indicator of the risk and presence of overweight in adolescents. Am J Clin Nutr 1999;70(suppl):131S–136S.
5   Baumgartner RN: Electrical impedance and total electrical body conductivity; in Roche AF, Heymsfield SB, Lohmann TG (eds): Human Body Composition. Human Kinetics, Champaign, 1996; pp 79–107.
6   Swan PD, McConnell KE: Anthropometry and bioelectrical impedance inconsistently predicts fatness in women with regional adiposity. Med Sci Sports Exerc 1999;31:1068–1075.
7   Möller R, Tafeit E, Smolle KH, Kullnig P: Lipometer: Determining the thickness of a subcutaneous fatty layer. Biosens Bioelectron 1994;9:xiii–xvi.
8   Möller R, Tafeit E, Smolle KH, Pieber TR, Ipsiroglu O, Duesse M, Huemer C, Sudi K, Reibnegger G: Estimating total body fat percentage and determining subcutaneous adipose tissue distribution with the non-invasive optical device Lipometer. Am J Hum Biol 2000;12:221–230.

9 Möller R, Tafeit E, Pieber TR, Sudi K, Reibnegger G: The measurement of subcutaneous adipose tissue topography (SAT-Top) by means of the new optical device LIPOMETER and the evaluation of standard factor coefficients for healthy subjects. Am J Hum Biol 2000;12:231–239.

10 Malina RM: Regional body composition: Age, sex, and ethnic variation; in Roche AF, Heymsfield SB, Lohmann TG (eds): Human Body Composition. Human Kinetics, Champaign, 1996, pp 217–255.

11 Schaefer F, Georgi M, Zieger A, Scharer K: Usefulness of bioelectric impedance and skinfold measurements in predicting fat-free mass derived from total body potassium in children. Pediatr Res 1994;35:617–624.

12 Malina RM, Bouchard C: Subcutaneous fat distribution during growth; in Bouchard C, Johnston FE (eds): Fat Distribution During Growth and Later Health Outcomes. New York, Plenum, 1988, pp 63–84.

Dr. Karl Sudi, Institute for Sport Sciences, Karl-Franzens University,
Mozartgasse 14, A–8010 Graz (Austria)
Tel. +43 316 380 2334, Fax +43 316 380 9790, E-Mail karl.sudi@kfunigraz.ac.at

Jürimäe T, Hills AP (eds): Body Composition Assessment in Children and Adolescents.
Med Sport Sci. Basel, Karger, 2001, vol 44, pp 46–52

....

Prediction Equations for the Determination of Body Composition in Children Using Bioimpedance Analysis

Vaclav Bunc

Faculty of Physical Education and Sports, Charles University, Prague,
Czech Republic

The measurement of body composition has become an important procedure in nutrition and health-oriented assessments. Dependent upon the subjects and the desired outcome various components of body composition can be assessed using a range of available methods. Despite recent advances in technology and the subsequent availability of relatively new techniques such as neutron-activation and computer tomography-scanning, the most frequently used body composition methods are still based on the results of the chemical and anthropological analysis of a limited number of human cadavers [1, 2]. From these analyses, three basic measurement techniques were established and accepted as reference methods. These methods include the densitometric technique, the dilution method for total body water, and the measurement of total body potassium (^{40}K) [3]. Each approach is based on a set of assumptions that are only valid for groups of healthy adults and are known to be invalid for many other groups [4–6]. Numerous 'indirect' and 'doubly indirect' methods have been derived from these reference methods. These include hydrostatic weighing – HW [7], skinfold thickness measurements – SF [7, 8] and bioimpedance analysis – BIA [9].

BIA is an attractive body composition methodology because the method is quick, easy, and noninvasive. The method may also be used on-line and is reliable and applicable for trained or untrained subjects or various patient groups of various ages [10]. Like most methods for the assessment of body composition, bioelectrical impedance depends upon several assumptions regarding the composition of the fat and the fat-free body. These include constancy in the relationships among these body compartments. However, the level of hydration and the density of the fat-free mass are not constant among individuals and vary as a function of age, race, gender and physical condition [11]. Such variability affects the general application of the technique and may confuse the interpretation of BIA results.

Impedance measurements in a biological system such as the human body are a function of the current frequency. This functional relationship is expressed in the reactance measure of impedance. At low frequencies, the bioelectrical current primarily passes through extracellular fluids and reactance is minimised since the capacitant properties are bypassed. At high frequencies, the current penetrates all body tissues completely and again, reactance is minimised as the high frequency prevents capacitant effects from occurring in the body tissues.

The majority of the commercial BIA analysers use the single frequency of 50 kHz. The choice of this frequency is based on the earlier work of Nyboer [12] who determined that this was the critical frequency of muscle tissue, the frequency at which maximum reactance occurs. Impedance measures of the human body at frequencies other than 50 kHz was first advanced by Thomasett's group [13] in the 1960s. This research group determined that measures of BIA at low and high frequencies could differentiate the proportion of extracellular fluid volume in the body.

The single-frequency BIA estimates of body composition assume that the total conductive volume of the body is equivalent to that of total body water and that the hydration of adipose tissue is minimal [14]. However, these relationships are not constant among individuals or groups of individuals. Therefore, whole-body measures of impedance, resistance, and reactance at 50 kHz are frequently used in combination with anthropometry to improve predictions of body composition by increasing the amount of shared variance among the dependent and independent variables.

The measurement accuracy and thus the use of BIA for body composition assessment is directly related to the prediction equation used [6]. During the last 15 years, numerous studies have resulted in the development of equations to predict body composition from impedance in children [15–21]. In these predictions, the dependent variable, either FFM or percent body fat, is derived from densitometry, total body water by deuterium dilution and dual-energy X-ray absorptiometry (DXA).

The independent variables most commonly used are height^{2*} resistance, body mass, gender and age. The term height^{2*} resistance is used because it is proportional to FFM. Body mass is correlated with FFM so that the inclusion of body mass with a positive regression coefficient is to be expected.

The problems inherent in the application of prediction equations to other samples as demonstrated in cross validation of selected equations, can be attributed to several factors [10]. The accuracy of a prediction depends on the validity of the measurement of the dependent variable and on the model of body composition used.

In the Czech population, prediction equations for the determination of body composition are lacking. Therefore, the purpose of this study was to determine the prediction equations for body composition determination in children using hydrostatic weight and/or DXA as the reference methods.

Subjects and Methods

A total of 213 children (122 boys and 91 girls) ranging in age from 6 to 15 years comprised the study population. The mean age of boys was 11.8 ± 3.6 years, and body mass, 36.8 ± 10.9 kg. The mean value for height was 147.4 ± 8.4 cm, percent body fat (% BF) was $17.0 \pm 5.6\%$, and FFM, 30.5 ± 6.2 cm. For girls, the mean age was 11.6 ± 3.9 years, and body mass, 38.4 ± 9.6 kg. Height for girls was 149.1 ± 5.6 cm, percent body fat was $22.0 \pm 6.1\%$, and FFM 30.0 ± 6.3 kg.

For the cross-validation of the determined prediction equations with % BF, a group of 45 children ranging in age from 7 to 15 years were assessed by hydrostatic weighing (HW). In a further group of 12 subjects, the % BF was higher using both the HW and the DXA method.

Whole-body impedance was measured using a commercially available bioimpedance system, the Bodystat 500 (Bodystat Ltd., Isle of Man, British Isles) and/or BIA 2000–M (Datainput, Frankfurt, Germany) by a tetrapolar electrode configuration in a supine position on the right hand and foot. Four electrodes were placed on each subject. A current-injecting electrode was placed on the dorsum of the right hand, 1 cm proximal to the knuckle at the base of the middle finger. The second current-injecting electrode was placed on the dorsum of the right foot, 2 cm proximal to the space between the large and second toe. The two voltage-sensing electrodes were placed midway between radial and ulnar tubercles and lateral and medial malleoli, respectively. Prior to positioning of the electrodes, each electrode site was prepared by swabbing with alcohol and then allowing the site to dry. An excitation current of 400 (BIA 2000–M) or 800 µA at a fixed 50 kHz frequency was introduced to the subject.

Body density was assessed by HW and/or DXA. The majority of the children (78%) were evaluated using HW. Hydrostatic weight was completed with a correction for residual lung volume using the oxygen dilution method of Wilmore [22]. Residual volume was determined on land with the subject seated in a position similar to that assumed during HW. Percent body fat was estimated from body density using the revised formula of Brozek et al. [23]. Determination of body fat percent by DXA was undertaken according to Clark et al. [2].

For the BIA prediction equations, the variables considered were the anthropometric parameters (height, height^2, body mass, body mass^2, age) and resistance (height^{2*} resistance^{-1}). Variables were entered automatically in the order in which they contributed to the prediction equation and were included in the final equation only if they resulted in a significant increase in the r^2 values or a significant reduction in the S_{EE}. Total error of estimate (T_{EE}) was calculated according to formula $TEE = \{(\text{Predicted \% BF} - \text{Actual \% BF})^2/n\}^{1/2}$. A repeated-measures ANOVA was used to test the differences between methods. Significance was determined at the 0.01% level.

Results

There were no significant differences in resistance between the Bodystat 500 and BIA 2000–M instruments at the frequency of 50 kHz. Similarly, there were no significant differences between % BF values determined by HW and DXA. According to the results of the present study, the critical age for % BF determination is 10 years. Therefore, different prediction equations are required for children younger than 10 years and over 10 years of age and up to 15 years. Adolescents older than 15 years of age may use equations developed for adults.

The prediction equation for % BF determination in boys under 10 years of age:

$$\% \ BF = 39.2649 - 5.4577*age \ (years) - 9.2044*Ht(m)^2 + 0.4177*mass(kg) + \\ + 0.0442*BIA(\Omega)$$
$$(r = 0.796, \ p < 0.001, \ S_{EE} = 0.94\%, \ T_{EE} = 1.06\%)$$

The prediction equation for % BF determination in girls under 10 years old:

$$\% \ BF = 14.6812 - 0.1105*age(years) + 0.5938*mass(kg) - 4.9063*Ht^2(m)*BIA^{-1}(\Omega)$$
$$(r = 0.748, \ p < 0.001, \ S_{EE} = 1.53\%, \ T_{EE} = 1.28\%)$$

The prediction equation for the older boys, 10.1–15 years:

$$\% \ BF = 6.4649 - 0.0577*age(years) - 9.2044*Ht(m)2 + 0.4077*mass(kg) + \\ + 0.0084*BIA^{-1}(\Omega)$$
$$(r = 0.809, \ p < 0.001, \ S_{EE} = 0.91\%, \ T_{EE} = 0.99\%)$$

The prediction equation for the older girls, 10.1–15 years:

$$\% \ BF = 10.8852 - 0.0968*age(years) + 0.5634*mass(kg) - 5.0603*Ht2(m)*BIA^{-1}(\Omega)$$
$$(r = 0.768, \ p < 0.001, \ S_{EE} = 1.33\%, \ T_{EE} = 1.18\%)$$

No significant differences were found between values of % BF determined by the equations presented above and values in the group of 45 children who were assessed by HW.

Discussion

The measurement of the electrical impedance between the wrist and ankle in human subjects is used extensively as a method of assessing body composition. However, Elsen et al. [25] identified two basic sources of error with BIA measurements, instrument error (the instrument's accuracy for measuring resistance), and measurement error, such as biological variation, electrode placement, and inter-observer variation. Apart from sources of error related to hardware, electrode placement also appears to be a major problem. For example, Elsen et al. [25] moved the sensor electrode proximally in 2 mm increments up the arm, up the leg and on both the arm and leg simultaneously until the electrode had been displaced a distance of 1 cm from the standard location. Changes in resistance were similar (2.1%) when the electrode was moved on the arm and then the leg. At a maximal displacement of 2 cm the change in resistance was 4.1%. When impedance was measured with the electrodes in the standard position, the coefficient of variation for repeated measurements was 0.4%. Additionally, no effects were observed for changes in the respiratory cycle. The authors conclude that thermoregulation and skin temperature may play a role in achieving accurate and precise impedance measurements. For the precise determination of BIA, one must try to define the hydration status of the subjects.

According to Lohman [26], the mean values for actual % BF (HW or DXA) and predicted % BF should be comparable. Similarly, a low S_{EE} value is desirable and is preferred over the correlation coefficient since the correlation is likely to be affected by inter-sample variability in % BF. T_{EE} should be calculated because it reflects the true differences between the actual and predicted % BF values, whereas S_{EE} only reflects error associated with regression between the variables. The S_D values for the actual and predicted % BF values should be in close agreement.

Both the S_{EE} (range from 0.91% to 1.53%) and the T_{EE} (range from 0.99% to 1.28%) were lower than the 3.8% level conventionally considered an acceptable error for field methods [26]. The differences between mean values of % BF determined by prediction equation for BIA and by SF and HW were nonsignificant. Additionally, values determined by means of BIA highly correlated with SF and HW and/or DXA values. This finding is consistent with other studies [27, 28].

No indirect error-free method currently exists to determine % BF. Indeed, the S_{EE} involved in the prediction of DXA % BF from body fat by BIA does not include the error associated with densitometry due to the variability in the density of the fat-free mass. The criterion method of HW has a reported error of 2.5% [26]. Thus, any method used is hampered by the lack of an accurate in vivo reference method. Each of the techniques used in this study can be affected by technical and biological errors. Although these errors were controlled as much as possible, certain assumptions (for example, absolute constancy of the chemical composition of the fat-free mass) are difficult to account for. The establishment of population-specific equations for BIA may further improve the accuracy of these methods.

In conclusion, BIA is a valid method for assessing body composition in children. The equations supplied by the manufacturers of the BIA devices must be adapted for specific groups of subjects. As there are no universally accepted equations for subjects with % BF in the range 3–30%, and in the age range of 6–60 years, appropriate age and % BF equations must be developed.

References

1   Widdowson EM, McCance R, Spray CM: The chemical composition of the human body. Clin Sci 1951;10:113–125.
2   Clarys JP, Marfell-Jones MJ: Soft tissue of the body and fractionation of the upper and lower limbs. Ergonomics 1994;37:217–229.
3   Forbes BG: Human Body Composition. New York, Springer, 1987.
4   Slaughter MH, Lohman TG, Boileau RA, Horswill CA, Stillman RJ, Van Loan MD, Bemben DA: Skinfold equations for estimation of body fatness in children and youth. Hum Biol 1988;60:709–723.
5   Deurenberg P, Leenen R, Van Der Kooy K, Hautvast JGAJ: In obese subjects the body fat percentage calculated with Siri's formula is an overestimation. Eur J Clin Nutr 1989;43:569–575
6   Deurenberg P, Werterterp KR, Velthuis-TeWierik EJM: Between-laboratory comparison of densito-metry and biomedical measurements. Br J Nutr 1994;1:309–316.
7   Siri WE: Body composition from fluid spaces and density: analysis of methods; in Brozek J, Henschel A (eds): Techniques for Measuring Body Composition. Washington, National Academy of Sciences, 1961, pp 223–244.
8   Durnin JVGA, Womersley J: Body fat assessed from total body density and its estimation from skinfold thickness: Measurements of 481 men and women aged from 17 to 72 years. Br J Clin Nutr 1974;32:77–97.
9   Parizkova J: Body Fat and Physical Fitness. Hague, Nijhoff, 1977.
10   Chumlea WC, Guo SS: Bioelectrical impedance and body composition: Present status and future directions. Nutr Rev 1994;52:123–131.
11   Lohman TG: Applicability of body composition techniques and constants for children and youths. Exerc Sport Sci Rev 1986;14:325–357.
12   Nyboer J: Electrical Impedance Plethysmography. Springfield, Thomas, 1959.
13   Thomasset A: Bio-electrical properties of tissue impedance measurement. Lyon Med 1962;217: 107–118.
14   Lukaski HC: (1987) Methods for the assessment of body composition: traditional and new. Am J Clin Nutr 1987;46:437–356.
15   Conlisk EA, Haas JD, Martinez EJ, Flores R, Rivera JD, Martonell R: Predicting body composition from anthropometry and bioimpedance in marginally undernourished adolescents and young adults. Am J Clin Nutr 1992;55:1051–1059.
16   Cordain L, Whicker RE, Johnson JE: Body composition determination in children using bioelectrical impedance. Growth Dev Aging 1988;52:37–40.
17   Davies PSW, Preece MA, Hicks CJ, Halliday D: The prediction of total body water using bioelectrical impedance in children and adolescents. Ann Hum Biol 1988;15:267–240.
18   Houtkooper LB, Lohman TG, Going SC, Hall MC: Validity of bioelectric impedance for body composition assessment in children. J Appl Physiol 1989;66:814–821.
19   Deurenberg P, Kooy KVD, Paling A, Withagen P: Assessment of body composition in 8–11 year old children by bioelectrical impedance. Eur J Clin Nutr 1989;43:623–629.
20   Deurenberg P, Kusters CSL, Smit HE: Assessment of body composition by bioelectrical impedance in children and young adults is strongly age-dependent. Eur J Clin Nutr 1990;44:261–268.

21 Deurenberg P, Kooy K, Leenen R, Weststrate JA, Seidell JC: Sex and age specific prediction formulas for estimating body composition from bioelectric impedance: A cross-validation study. Int J Obes 1991;15:17–25.

22 Wilmore JHA: A simplified method for determination of residual lung volume. J Appl Physiol 1969; 27:96–100.

23 Brozek J, Grande F, Anderson JT, Keys A: Densitometric analysis of body composition: revision of some quantitative assumption. Ann NY Acad Sci 1963;110:113–140.

24 Clark RR, Kuta JM, Sullivan JC: Prediction of percent body fat in adult males using dual x-ray absorptiometry, skinfolds, and hydrostatic weighing. Med Sci Sports Exerc 1993;25:528–535.

25 Elsen R, Siu ML, Pineda O, Solomons NW: Sources of variability in bioelectrical impedance determinations in adults; in Ellis KJ (ed): In vivo Body Composition Studies. London, Inst Phys Sci Med, 1987, pp 184–188.

26 Lohman TG: Skinfold and body density and their relation to body fatness: A review. Hum Biol 1981;53:181–225.

27 Eaton AW, Israel RG, O'Brien KF, Hortobagyi T: Comparison of four methods to assess body composition in women. Eur J Clin Nutr 1993;47:353–360.

28 Stout RJ, Eckerson JM, Housh TJ, Johnson GO, Betts NM: Validity of percent body fat estimation in males. Med Sci Sports Exerc 1994;26:632–636.

Prof. Dr. Vaclav Bunc, PhD, Faculty of Physical Education and Sports,
Charles University, J. Martiho 31, CZ–162 52 Prague 6 (Czech Republic)
Tel./Fax +42 02 2017 2288

Jürimäe T, Hills AP (eds): Body Composition Assessment in Children and Adolescents.
Med Sport Sci. Basel, Karger, 2001, vol 44, pp 53–60

....

Whole Body Resistance Measured between Different Limbs and Resistance Indices in Pre-Adolescent Children

J. Jürimäe, A. Leppik, T. Jürimäe

Institute of Sport Pedagogy, University of Tartu, Estonia

As in adults [1], the measurement of body composition in children [2, 3] using bioelectrical impedance analysis (BIA) has utilised the resistance index (RI) in different equations (RI = stature^2/R). Houtkooper et al. [4] reported that RI, in conjunction with body mass, accurately predicted fat-free mass (FFM) in children aged 10–14 years. Danford et al. [5] indicated that RI was the single most significant predictor of total body water, accounting for 97% of the total variability in 5- to 9-year-old healthy children. However, Delozier et al. [6] reported that stature and body mass were better predictors of total body water than RI in children aged 4–8 years. Probably the squaring the stature of 'short' subjects did not result in as large a range of values for the resistance index.

Stature is not the true conductor length when using the four-electrode wrist-to-ankle method of BIA [7]. The true length of the conductor could be better represented by the sum of acromial stature and the arm length, and the total body impedance has a stronger predictor value than the segmental impedance measurements of the arm, leg and trunk do in adults [8].

Recently, the measurement of body impedance across both lower extremities (leg-to-leg) has been incorporated into a single frequency (50 kHz) BIA system (Tanita TBF 105, Tanita Corp, Tokyo, Japan). The leg-to-leg pressure contact electrode apparatus has been presented [9]. The body resistance between hands have also been measured (OMRON). There is a lack of information about the differences on the body resistance measured traditionally between arm-to-leg on the right side of the body or on the left side of the body or between lower and upper extremities in children. We hypothesised that the best possibility is to measure between the right leg and left hand or between left leg and right hand for the true measurement of body resistance. Secondly, we hypothesised that stature is not a correct length of the conductor (body) and it is better to use our presented equations where the 'true' length of the conductor (body) is used. The aim of this study was to compare the results of body resistance measured at different sites of the body in pre-adolescent children.

Methods

The subjects for this investigation were 104 boys and 105 girls, 9–11 years of age. The children were from several schools in Tartu (Estonia). The children participated in 2–3 compulsory physical education lessons per week at school. All children, parents and teachers were thoroughly informed about the purposes and contents of the study and written informed consent was obtained from the parents before participation. The study was approved by the Medical Ethics Committee of the University of Tartu (Estonia).

All measurements were performed in the morning at school after emptying the bladder. All children had a light traditional breakfast, and did not exercise before the testing. All children were on Tanner stage 1 [10]. Therefore, the children were classified prepubertal as pubic hair and genitalia (boys), and breast (girls) ratings were both scored as stage 1.

Stature was measured using a Martin metal anthropometer in cm (± 0.1 cm) and body mass with medical scales in kg (± 0.05 kg). BMI (kg/m^2) was also calculated. Anthropometric measurements were taken by a trained anthropometrist who had previously shown test-retest reliability of $r > 0.90$. The CENTURION KIT instrumentation was used (Rosscraft, Surrey, BC, Canada). The following parameters were measured: acromial stature, acromiale-radiale and radiale-stylion length both on right and left side, trochanterion-tibiale laterale and tibiale mediale-sphyrion tibiale segments length, biacromial breadth and biiliocristal breath. Additionally, the trunk diameters between trochanterion and acromiale were measured on both sides of the body. All anthropometric variables were measured according to the protocol recommended by the International Society for the Advancement of Kinanthropometry [11].

Body resistance was measured using a multiple-frequency impedance device (Multiscan 5000, Bodystat Ltd., UK). Children were placed on a table in a supine position with the limbs slightly abducted. Skin current electrodes were placed on the dorsal surface of the hand and foot at the metacarpals and metatarsals. The distance between the source and the receiving electrodes was greater than 5 cm at all times [12]. The Multiscan 5000 operates at a normal current of 200 µA at frequencies from 5 to 500 kHz. Data at all frequencies (5–500 kHz) were analysed, but only a part of the results is presented – 5 kHz as a measure of extracellular water, 50 kHz as a measure of total body water and 200 kHz as a measure of intracellular water. Body resistance of electric current was measured on the right side of the body followed by the measurement on the left side of the body. Resistance was also measured between hands and legs, and diagonally between right hand and left leg, and left hand and right leg of the body. Additionally, the RI was calculated using the traditional method: stature^2 divided by the body resistance at 50 kHz measured on the right and left side of the body, and also measured between hands and legs, and diagonally between right hand and left leg and right leg and left hand of the body. The new RI were calculated where the 'true' length of the conductor squared divided by the body resistance at 50 kHz. The following 'true' lengths of the conductor were used: acromial stature plus acromiale-radiale and radiale stylion length both on the right and left side; trunk diameter plus right hand and left leg length and trunk diameter plus left hand and right leg length; trochanterion-tibiale laterale and tibiale mediale-sphyrion tibiale segments length both on the right and left side plus biiliocristal breath.

Standard statistical methods were used to calculate mean ($\bar{X}$) and standard deviation ($\pm SD$). Statistical comparisons between boys and girls were made using independent t-tests. Spearman correlation coefficients were used to determine the relationships between dependent variables. Significance was set at $p \leq 0.05$.

Results

Boys were older (10.09 ± 0.84 and 9.79 ± 0.72 years) and their body weight (35.27 ± 5.71 and 33.29 ± 6.43 kg) and BMI (17.07 ± 1.78 and 16.50 ± 2.15) were significantly ($p < 0.05$) higher than in girls. There were no statistically significant ($p > 0.05$) differences between the sexes in stature (143.39 ± 7.27 and 141.49 ± 7.34 cm, respectively).

The mean body resistance measured at different sites is presented in table 1. In all cases, mean resistance was significantly higher in girls in comparison with boys ($p < 0.001$). The mean difference between right and left side measurements at 50 kHz was 16.6Ω (2.8%) and 17.2Ω (2.7%) in boys and girls, respectively. The body resistance measured diagonally (right hand-left leg or left hand-right leg) was similar and comparable with right and left side measurements ($p > 0.05$). However, the resistance measured between hands was significantly ($p < 0.001$) higher and resistance measured between legs significantly lower ($p < 0.01$–0.001) in comparison with the measurements of the other sites.

The relationships between body resistance measured in different sites in boys and girls are presented in table 2. The Spearman correlations were higher than $r = 0.80$ except between hands and legs ($r = 0.53$) in boys. In girls, the relationships between different measurement sites were slightly lower.

The mean resistance indices calculated using the traditional equations (S^2/R), or using the 'true' length of the conductor are presented in table 3. The mean indices were significantly higher in boys than in girls ($p < 0.001$). There were not any statistically significant differences between the indices calculated on the right or left side or diagonally ($p > 0.05$). However, the mean indices were lower when measured between hands and higher when measured between legs ($p < 0.05$–0.001).

Table 1. Body resistance measured at different sites

	5 kHz	50 kHz	200 kHz
Right side			
Boys	622.4 ± 65.0	578.8 ± 58.3	522.8 ± 53.6
Girls	671.1 ± 68.9	626.8 ± 56.6	564.2 ± 50.6
Left side			
Boys	637.5 ± 66.0	595.4 ± 61.3	540.8 ± 58.5
Girls	692.9 ± 69.4	644.0 ± 60.6	587.3 ± 54.0
Hand-hand			
Boys	687.8 ± 74.4	650.3 ± 71.0	592.6 ± 65.2
Girls	759.9 ± 83.6	713.5 ± 72.5	653.3 ± 64.6
Leg-leg			
Boys	525.9 ± 53.5	485.1 ± 48.9	439.1 ± 47.3
Girls	581.3 ± 61.9	532.5 ± 60.0	480.5 ± 58.2
Right hand-left leg			
Boys	635.8 ± 67.3	592.7 ± 60.4	539.2 ± 55.8
Girls	711.1 ± 72.8	657.5 ± 65.0	595.9 ± 59.9
Left hand-right leg			
Boys	632.4 ± 68.1	592.4 ± 61.7	539.2 ± 57.1
Girls	702.8 ± 69.5	650.8 ± 62.6	593.3 ± 51.6

Table 2. Relationship between body resistance measured in different sites

	Right side		Left side		Hand-hand		Leg-leg		Right hand-left leg		Left hand-right leg	
	boys	girls	boys	girls	boys	girls	boys	girls	boys	girls	boys	girls
Right side												
Left side	0.88	0.89										
Hand-hand	0.82	0.84	0.84	0.83								
Leg-leg	0.84	0.59	0.87	0.60	0.53	0.43						
Right hand-left leg	0.87	0.78	0.88	0.76	0.85	0.82	0.83	0.67				
Left hand-right leg	0.86	0.78	0.89	0.74	0.88	0.80	0.82	0.63	0.88	0.79		

Table 3. Mean resistance indices (S^2/R) measured in different sites

	Boys (n = 104)	Girls (n = 105)	p
Right side			
Old	36.14 ± 5.20	32.98 ± 5.14	<0.001
New	43.28 ± 7.28	38.40 ± 7.81	<0.001
Left side			
Old	35.27 ± 7.03	31.35 ± 5.03	<0.001
New	42.57 ± 8.63	37.60 ± 6.89	<0.001
Hand-hand			
Old	32.25 ± 5.18	28.60 ± 5.49	<0.001
New	30.04 ± 5.28	26.07 ± 4.92	<0.001
Leg-leg			
Old	43.22 ± 7.08	39.22 ± 6.70	<0.001
New	52.33 ± 10.46	48.56 ± 9.87	<0.001
Right hand-left leg			
Old	35.12 ± 5.64	31.22 ± 5.69	<0.001
New	45.08 ± 7.85	40.35 ± 7.64	<0.001
Left hand-right leg			
Old	35.06 ± 5.49	31.37 ± 5.15	<0.001
New	45.52 ± 7.79	40.96 ± 7.81	<0.001

The relationships between resistance indices calculated between different sites using traditional and new equations in boys and girls are presented in table 4. As a rule, the correlation coefficients were similar in boys and girls. Surprisingly, the relationships between hands and legs were the same as on the other sites.

Discussion

Mean body resistance of children in the current study was comparable with the results of other studies where 10- to 14-year-old children were measured [4]. Similarly, the difference between right and left side measurements was statistically significant (p < 0.001). Graves et al. [13] also noted that the resistance is systematically greater on the left side than on the right side by about 8 Ω. Thus, the side on which resistance is measured must be the side where body resistance was measured during the development of the body composition

---

Table 4. Relationship between resistance indices calculated between different sites using traditional and new equations

	Right side		Left side		Hand-hand		Leg-leg		Right hand-left leg		Left hand-right leg	
	boys	girls	boys	girls	boys	girls	boys	girls	boys	girls	boys	girls
Right side												
Left side												
Old	0.74	0.96										
New	0.76	0.88										
Hand-hand												
Old	0.92	0.88	0.82	0.85								
New	0.93	0.83	0.80	0.90								
Leg-leg												
Old	0.92	0.94	0.83	0.97	0.89	0.81						
New	0.89	0.83	0.81	0.93	0.83	0.86						
Right hand-left leg												
Old	0.91	0.80	0.82	0.80	0.95	0.75	0.96	0.78				
New	0.89	0.86	0.81	0.93	0.91	0.96	0.86	0.93				
Left hand-right leg												
Old	0.92	0.90	0.83	0.89	0.95	0.83	0.96	0.88	0.97	0.74		
New	0.93	0.73	0.84	0.79	0.93	0.86	0.91	0.86	0.94	0.90		

predictive equation. There were no statistically significant ($p > 0.05$) differences between resistance values while measured on the right side or diagonally (i.e. right hand-left leg or left hand-right leg) of the body. Thus, our results did not confirm our first hypothesis that it is better to measure body resistance diagonally between hand and opposite leg than on the right side of the body. It was concluded that the measurement of body resistance on the right side of the body is correct in pre-adolescent children.

The lower and upper body resistances are higher than whole body resistance (right arm-trunk-right leg) because of the relatively smaller volumes of these body segments in comparison with the trunk [14]. In the present study, the resistance between hands at 50 kHz was significantly higher when measured between legs. One of the explanations could be that the breadths of the hands are slightly shorter than of the legs. It is well known that thinner segments of the body provide greatest resistance [13–16].

The use of traditional resistance indices (S^2/R) for calculation of body composition is questionnable. Most researchers confirm that the presented indices (RI) is applicable for the calculation of different body composition parameters [1, 3, 17, 18]. However, some researchers [6] have recommended additional anthropometric variables to stature be used in equations. The main problem is that stature is not the correct length of the conductor. For example, Chumlea et al. [12] indicated that the use of shoulder height plus arm length rather than stature as a measure of the length of the conductor improves the accuracy of prediction marginally. Nunez et al. [9] have recommended that leg length be used as an electrical path length when using the leg-to-leg system. In our study, the real lengths of the conductors were measured and squared, and finally divided by the body resistance at 50 kHz. The use of a new RI needs further investigation as the RI was not compared with a direct measure of TBW in the present study.

In conclusion, this study indicates that the measurement of body resistance on the right side of the body is correct. The use of leg-to-leg or hand-to-hand electrodes needs additional validation. Probably, the use of a new RI where the 'true' length of the conductor is used, is more correct than the traditional approach where stature is used.

Acknowledgements

We wish to express our thanks to Professors Albrecht Claessens and Han Kemper for their comments and suggestions.

References

1   Lohman TG: Advances in body composition assessment. Current issues in exercise science series. Monograph No 3. Champaign, Human Kinetics, 1992.
2   Davies PSW, Preece MA, Hicks CJ, Halliday D: The prediction of total body water using bioelectrical impedance in children and adolescents. Ann Hum Biol 1988;15:237–240.
3   Kuschner RF: Bioelectrical impedance analysis: A review of principles and applications. J Am Coll Nutr 1992;11:199–209.
4   Houtkooper LB, Lohman TG, Going SB, Hall MC: Validity of bioelectric impedance for body composition assessment in children. J Appl Physiol 1989;66:814–821.
5   Danford LC, Schoeller DA, Kushner RF: Comparison of two bioelectrical impedance analysis models for total body water measurement in children. Ann Hum Biol 1992;19:603–607.
6   Delozier MG, Gutin B, Wang J, Basch CE, Contento I, Shea S, Irioyen M, Zybert P, Rips J, Pierson R: Validity of anthropometry and bioimpedance with 4– to 8–year-olds using total body water as the criterion. Pediatr Exerc Sci 1991;3:238–249.
7   Baumgartner RN, Chumlea WC, Roche AF: Bioelectric impedance for body composition. Exerc Sport Sci Rev 1990;18:193–224.
8   Grieve C, Henneberg M: Statistical significance of body impedance measurements in estimating body composition. Homo 1998;49:1–12.

9   Nunez C, Callagher D, Visser M, Xavier Pi-Sunyer F, Wang Z, Heymsfield SB: Bioimpedance analysis: Evaluation of leg-to-leg system based on pressure contact foot-pad electrodes. Med Sci Sports Exerc 1997;29:524–531.
10   Tanner JM: Growth at Adolescence, ed 2. Oxford, Blackwell Scientific, 1962.
11   Norton KI, Whittingham N, Carter JEL, Kerr D, Gore C, Marfell-Jones MJ: Measurement techniques in anthropometry; in Norton KI, Olds TS (eds): Anthropometrica. Sydney, UNSW Press, 1996, pp 25–75.
12   Chumlea WC, Baumgartner RN, Roche AF: The use of specific resistivity used to estimate fat free mass from segmental body measures of bioelectric impedance. Am J Clin Nutr 1988;48:7–15.
13   Graves JE, Pollock ML, Colvin AB, Van Loan M, Lohman TG: Comparison of different bioelectrical impedance analyzers in the prediction of body composition. Am J Hum Biol 1989;1:603–612.
14   Heyward VH: Practical body composition assessment for children, adults and older adults. Int J Sport Nutr 1998;8:285–307.
15   Fuller NJ, Elia M: Potential use of bioelectric impedance of the 'whole body' and of body segments for the assessment of body composition: Comparison with densitometry. Eur J Clin Nutr 1989;43: 779–791.
16   Baumgartner RN, Chumlea WC, Roche AF: Associations between bioelectrical impedance and anthropometric variables. Hum Biol 1987;59:235–244.
17   Lukaski HC, Johnson PE, Bolonchuk WW, Lykken GI: Assessment of fat-free mass using bioelectric impedance measurements of the human body. Am J Clin Nutr 1985;41:810–817.
18   Hoffer ED, Meador CK, Simpson DC: Correlation of whole-body impedance with total body water. J Appl Physiol 1969;27:531–534.

Dr. Jaak Jürimäe, PhD, University of Tartu, 18 Ülikooli Street, 51014 Tartu (Estonia)
Tel. +372 7 375 372, Fax +372 7 375 373 E-Mail jaakj@ut.ee

Jürimäe T, Hills AP (eds): Body Composition Assessment in Children and Adolescents.
Med Sport Sci. Basel, Karger, 2001, vol 44, pp 61–70

....

Influence of Anthropometric Variables to the Whole-Body Resistance in Pre-Adolescent Children

T. Jürimäe, A. Leppik, J. Jürimäe

Institute of Sport Pedagogy, University of Tartu, Estonia

Bioelectrical impedance analysis (BIA) is a safe, portable, noninvasive, rapid and inexpensive method to determine body composition [1]. BIA is based upon the relationship between the volume of the conductor (i.e. the human body), the conductor's length, the components of the conductor and its impedance.

Total body impedance, measured at the constant frequency of 50 kHz (800 μA), primarily reflects the volumes of water and muscle compartments comprising the fat-free mass (FFM) and the extracellular water volume [2]. However, the intracellular penetration is not complete at this frequency. Differences in the distribution of fluid between intra-and extracellular compartments which occur during growth and development, could help explain the variability in the prediction of fluid status or change in fluid status in children.

The new impedance instruments are able to measure body impedance at more than one frequency, ranging from low (about 1 kHz) to very high (> 1 MHz) [3]. At low frequency, body impedance is a measure of extracellular water (ECW) and at high frequency body impedance is a measure of intracellular water (ICW). However, different segments of the body contribute to the resistance of the whole body to an extent that is out of proportion to their contribution to body weight [4, 5]. For example, the arm contributes only about 4% of body weight but as much as 45% to the resistance of the whole body in adults [4]. The thinner segments of the body provide the greatest resistance, especially when these segments are also long [4]. The influence of different anthropometric variables on the body resistance in children is poorly studied. However, the percentage of body water in boys from birth to 10 years

Table 1. Mean anthropometric variables in prepubertal children ($\bar{X} \pm SD$)

	Boys (n = 104)	Girls (n = 105)
Age, years	10.09 ± 0.84	9.79 ± 0.72*
Stature, cm	143.39 ± 7.27	141.49 ± 7.34
Body mass, kg	35.27 ± 5.71	33.29 ± 6.43*
BMI, kg/m²	17.07 ± 1.78	16.50 ± 2.15*
Skinfolds, mm		
Triceps	9.97 ± 3.01	11.17 ± 3.91*
Subscapular	7.33 ± 3.50	8.42 ± 5.06*
Biceps	6.63 ± 2.53	7.50 ± 3.38*
Iliac crest	8.67 ± 4.82	9.30 ± 5.46
Supraspinale	5.13 ± 2.65	6.20 ± 3.84
Abdominal	8.73 ± 5.07	9.67 ± 6.20
Front thigh	16.46 ± 5.59	18.02 ± 5.85
Medial calf	12.32 ± 4.49	13.32 ± 5.18
Mid axilla	5.40 ± 1.95	6.22 ± 3.65*
Girths, cm		
Head	53.25 ± 1.43	52.55 ± 1.56*
Neck	28.00 ± 1.87	26.74 ± 1.35*
Arm relaxed	20.08 ± 2.00	19.62 ± 2.32*
Arm flexed and tensed	21.70 ± 2.01	20.98 ± 2.36*
Forearm	19.79 ± 1.39	18.95 ± 1.57*
Wrist	13.58 ± 0.86	12.94 ± 0.81*
Chest	68.44 ± 4.66	65.98 ± 6.04*
Waist	59.96 ± 4.39	56.39 ± 5.08
Gluteal	71.62 ± 5.47	71.57 ± 6.31
Thigh	42.44 ± 4.15	42.40 ± 4.94
Thigh mid-troch-tibiale laterale	39.10 ± 3.52	38.99 ± 3.98
Calf	28.44 ± 2.37	28.25 ± 2.48
Ankle	18.66 ± 1.48	18.26 ± 1.41*
Length, cm		
Acromiale radiale	30.34 ± 1.80	30.02 ± 1.91
Radiale-stylion	22.88 ± 1.51	22.41 ± 1.50*
Midstylion-dactylion	16.64 ± 1.07	16.19 ± 1.06*
Iliospinale box height	82.67 ± 5.10	81.30 ± 4.88
Trochanterion box height	76.00 ± 4.61	74.94 ± 5.40
Trochanterion-tibiale laterale	38.94 ± 2.73	38.71 ± 2.85
Tibiale-laterale to floor	37.02 ± 2.54	36.48 ± 2.58
Tibiale mediale–sphyrion tibiale	29.33 ± 2.21	29.05 ± 2.06

Table 1 (continued)

	Boys (n = 104)	Girls (n = 105)
Breadths/length, cm		
Biacromial	31.76 ± 1.86	30.94 ± 2.03*
Biiliocristal	21.87 ± 1.56	21.88 ± 1.63
Foot length	22.32 ± 1.63	21.91 ± 1.30*
Sitting height	75.67 ± 3.57	74.46 ± 3.83*
Transverse chest	21.90 ± 2.59	20.73 ± 1.35
A-P chest depth	15.07 ± 2.19	14.42 ± 2.59*
Humerus	6.10 ± 0.38	5.82 ± 0.35*
Femur	8.82 ± 0.46	8.36 ± 0.47*

* Significantly different from boys: $p < 0.05$.

of age has been reported to decrease as does the ratio of extra- and intracellular water [6]. Variation in hydration of fat free mass (FFM) is relatively high in children [7]. The purpose of this study was to investigate the possible relationships between skinfold thickness, girth, length and breadth/length parameters and body resistance at different frequencies in 9- to 11-year-old children.

Methods

The subjects of this investigation were 104 boys and 105 girls, 9- to 11-years of age. The children were from several schools in Tartu, Estonia (about 100,000 inhabitants) and all children were of Estonian origin. School physical education consisted of 2–3 physical education lessons per week, taught by a physical education teacher. All children, parents and teachers were thoroughly informed about the purposes and contents of the study and written informed consent was obtained from the parents or the adult probands before participation. This study was approved by the Medical Ethics Committee of the University of Tartu (Estonia).

Measurements were performed in the morning at school after emptying the bladder. All children had a light traditional breakfast. The children did not exercise before the testing. All children were classified prepubertal Tanner stage 1 [8] as pubic hair and genitalia (boys), and breast (girls) ratings were both scored as stage 1.

Stature was measured using a Martin metal anthropometer in cm (± 0.1 cm) and body mass with medical scales in kg (± 0.05 kg) and BMI (kg/m²) was calculated. In total, nine skinfolds (triceps, subscapular, biceps, iliac crest, supraspinale, abdominal, front thigh, medial calf, mid-axilla), 13 girths (head, neck, arm relaxed, arm flexed and tensed, forearm, wrist, chest, waist, gluteal, thigh, thigh mid trochanter-tibiale laterale, calf, ankle), eight lengths (acromiale-radiale, radiale-stylion, midstylion-dactylion, iliospinale-box height, trochan-

Table 2. Relationships between anthropometric variables and body resistance in boys and girls

	Boys (n = 104)			Girls (n = 105)		
	5 kHz	50 kHz	200 kHz	5 kHz	50 kHz	200 kHz
Stature	NS	NS	NS	−0.20	−0.19	−0.16
Body mass	−0.44	−0.43	−0.41	−0.42	−0.42	−0.40
BMI	−0.47	−0.50	−0.51	−0.45	−0.45	−0.45
Skinfolds						
Triceps	NS	NS	NS	−0.30	−0.26	−0.26
Subscapular	NS	NS	NS	−0.21	−0.22	−0.22
Biceps	NS	NS	ŃS	−0.30	−0.25	−0.24
Iliac crest	−0.22	−0.20	−0.20	−0.26	−0.26	−0.25
Supraspinale	−0.23	−0.21	−0.20	−0.28	−0.26	−0.25
Abdominal	NS	NS	NS	−0.26	−0.22	−0.20
Front thigh	NS	NS	NS	−0.29	−0.29	−0.28
Medial calf	NS	NS	NS	−0.35	−0.30	−0.30
Mid-axilla	−0.23	−0.22	−0.22	−0.25	−0.23	−0.22
Girth						
Head	NS	NS	NS	NS	−0.19	NS
Neck	−0.49	−0.49	−0.48	−0.47	−0.49	−0.48
Arm relaxed	−0.52	−0.56	−0.57	−0.44	−0.45	−0.47
Arm flexed and tensed	−0.44	−0.53	−0.55	−0.46	−0.47	−0.49
Forearm	−0.54	−0.57	−0.57	−0.45	−0.45	−0.43
Wrist	−0.60	−0.60	−0.62	−0.46	−0.46	−0.44
Chest	−0.42	−0.45	−0.46	−0.38	−0.40	−0.39
Waist	−0.35	−0.38	−0.39	−0.36	−0.35	−0.35
Gluteal	−0.40	−0.41	−0.40	−0.44	−0.44	−0.44
Thigh	−0.40	−0.42	−0.41	−0.45	−0.44	−0.45
Thigh mid-troch-tibiale laterale	−0.43	−0.45	−0.45	−0.47	−0.48	−0.49
Calf	−0.48	−0.51	−0.51	−0.47	−0.47	−0.49
Ankle	−0.52	−0.53	−0.52	−0.48	−0.47	−0.46
Length						
Acromiale-radiale	NS	NS	NS	−0.22	−0.23	NS
Radiale-stylion	−0.30	−0.24	−0.21	NS	NS	NS
Midstylion-dactylion	−0.27	−0.23	−0.20	−0.24	−0.24	NS
Iliospinale box height	NS	NS	NS	−0.20	NS	NS
Trochanterion	NS	NS	NS	NS	NS	NS
Trochanterion-tibiale laterale	NS	NS	NS	NS	NS	NS
Tibiale-laterale to floor	NS	NS	NS	−0.21	NS	NS
Tibiale mediale sphyrion tibiale	NS	NS	NS	NS	NS	NS

Table 2 (continued)

Breadths/length	Boys (n = 104)			Girls (n = 105)		
	5 kHz	50 kHz	200 kHz	5 kHz	50 kHz	200 kHz
Biacromial	−0.38	−0.38	−0.37	−0.26	−0.26	−0.22
Biiliocristal	−0.29	−0.29	−0.28	NS	NS	NS
Foot length	−0.32	−0.30	−0.28	−0.22	−0.21	NS
Sitting height	−0.30	−0.28	−0.26	−0.20	−0.21	NS
Transverse chest	−0.24	−0.31	−0.33	−0.31	−0.32	−0.32
A-P chest depth	NS	NS	NS	−0.27	−0.27	−0.25
Humerus	−0.52	0.53	−0.53	−0.37	−0.38	−0.37
Femur	−0.41	−0.41	−0.40	−0.39	−0.36	−0.34

NS = Not significant.

terion-box height, trochanterion-tibiale laterale, tibiale-laterale to floor, tibiale mediale-sphyrion tibiale) and eight breadths/lengths (biacromial, biiliocristal, foot length, sitting height, transverse chest, A-P chest depth, humerus, femur) were measured. Three series of anthropometric measurements were taken by a trained anthropometrist who had previously shown test-retest reliability of r > 0.90. The CENTURION KIT instrumentation was used (Rosscraft, Surrey, BC, Canada). However, the skinfold thicknesses were measured using Holtain (Crymmych, UK) skinfold calipers. Calibration of all equipment was conducted prior to and at regular intervals during the data collection period. The nine measures of skinfold thicknesses were summed and the waist/hip and waist/thigh girth ratios were calculated. All anthropometric parameters were measured according to the protocol recommended by International Society for Advancement of Kinanthropometry [9].

The body resistance was measured with a multiple-frequency impedance device (MULTISCAN 5000, Bodystat Ltd., UK). Children were placed in a supine position with limbs slightly abduced. Skin current electrodes were placed on the right dorsal surface at the hand and on foot at the metacarpals and metatarsals, respectively after the skin was cleaned with 70% alcohol. The distance between the source and receiving electrodes was at all times greater than 5 cm [5]. All frequencies were analyzed, but only data at 5 kHz (as a measure of ECW), 50 kHz (as a measure of total body water [TBW]) and 200 kHz (as a measure of ICW) were used. The analyzer was calibrated before each test by using the standard resistor provided by the manufacturer. All measurements of children were performed on the same day and were completed within 1 h of the commencement of testing.

Standard statistical methods were used to calculate mean ($\bar{X}$) and standard deviation ($\pm$SD). Statistical comparisons between boys and girls were made using independent t-tests. Spearman correlation coefficients were used to determine the relationships between dependent variables. The effect of different anthropometric parameters on the body resistance was analyzed by stepwise multiple regression analysis. Prediction errors for the equations were evaluated using standard error of estimate (SEE). Significance was set at $p \le 0.05$.

Results

The mean data for anthropometric parameters of boys and girls are presented in table 1. Boys were older and their body mass and BMI were higher than in girls (p<0.05). The skinfold thicknesses on the triceps, subscapular, biceps and mid-axilla sites were significantly higher in girls (p<0.05). The sum of nine skinfold thicknesses was 80.3 ± 29.9 and 90.2 ± 39.7 mm in boys and in girls, respectively (p<0.05). There were no significant differences in the length parameters between boys and girls (except radiale stylion and midstylion-dactylion). Most of the measured breadth/length parameters and girths were higher in boys (p<0.05). The mean body resistance at 5, 50 and 200 kHz were 622.4 ± 65.0, 578.8 ± 58.3 and $522.8 \pm 53.6 \, \Omega$ in boys, respectively, and 671.1 ± 68.9, 626.8 ± 56.6 and $564.2 \pm 50.6 \, \Omega$, in girls, respectively. The resistance was significantly (p<0.01–0.001) higher in girls in comparison with boys.

The Spearman correlations between body resistance and different measured anthropometric parameters are presented in table 2. Stature significantly influenced body resistance in girls. For both genders, body weight and BMI were more important predictors. All skinfold thicknesses correlated significantly with body resistance in girls ($r=-0.20$ to 0.35), while only iliac crest, supraspinale and mid-axilla sites correlated significantly with body resistance in boys. The sum of skinfolds only correlated significantly with body resistance in girls ($r=-0.27$). As a rule, the girth parameters correlated significantly ($r=-0.19$ to -0.62) with body resistance in both boys and girls. The waist/hip girths ratio did not correlate significantly with body resistance. However, the relationship between waist/thigh ratio and body resistance was significant in boys ($r=0.24$) and girls ($r=0.35$). There were only a very few length parameters which influenced significantly body resistance. Most of the measured breadth/length parameters correlated significantly with body resistance but at relatively low level ($r=0.20–0.53$).

Stepwise multiple regression analysis indicated that girth parameters influenced the body resistance in boys (table 3). Wrist, neck, gluteal and relaxed arm girth characterized 51.2% of the total variance ($R^2 \times 100$). The importance of length and especially skinfold thicknesses was low. Wrist girth, front thigh skinfold thickness and arm (relaxed) girth characterized 47.4% of the total variance for all anthropometric parameters.

Girths (neck, arm flexed and tensed, waist) characterized 31.3% of the total variance in girls (table 4) with the medial calf responsible for 9.2% of the total variance from the measured skinfolds. The length parameters (acromiale-radiale) characterized only 5.1% of the total variance. In total, the anthropometric parameters used (arm flexed and tensed girth, subscapular

Table 3. Regression analysis of body resistance at 50 kHz with anthropometry in boys (n = 104)

	Intercept	F	R²×100	p	SEE
Skinfolds					
	613.9	5.1	4.8	<0.03	57.2
Mid-axilla	−6.5				
Girth					
	1,131.7	25.9	51.2	<0.0000	41.6
Wrist	−41.6				
Neck	−5.9				
Gluteal	6.7				
Arm-relaxed	−14.9				
Length					
	688.4	7.2	12.5	<0.0012	55.1
Radiale-stylion	−24.4				
Iliospinale	5.4				
Breadths/length					
	1,078.7	39.8	28.1	<0.0000	49.7
Humerus	−81.9				
Total					
	1,173.1	30.1	47.4	<0.0000	42.9
Wrist girth	−27.9				
Front thigh skinfold	3.7				
Arm (relaxed) girth	−13.7				

skinfold and tibiale-mediale length) characterized 32.1% of the total variance. SEE was relatively high in all presented regression equations.

Discussion

Theoretically, estimates of body composition from whole-body bioelectrical impedance have been based on the equation $V = p \times S^2/R$, in which conductive volume (V) is assumed to represent TBW or FFM, p is the specific resistivity of the conductor, stature (S) is taken as an estimate of the length of the conductor and R is a body impedance [1, 2, 5, 10]. However, probably stature is not a true conductor length when using the four-electrode wrist-to-ankle method of BIA. The true length of the conductor could be better

Table 4. Regression analysis of body resistance at 50 kHz with anthropometry in girls (n = 105)

	Intercept	F	R² × 100	p	SEE
Skinfolds					
	670.8	10.4	9.2	<0.002	54.2
Medial calf	−3.3				
Girth					
	1,096.0	15.4	31.3	<0.0000	47.6
Neck	−19.9				
Arm flexed and tensed	−14.9				
Waist	6.7				
Length					
	828.5	5.6	5.1	<0.02	55.4
Acromiale-radiale	−6.7				
Breadths/length					
	956.3	9.6	15.8	<0.0002	52.4
Transverse chest	−12.4				
A-P chest depth	−5.1				
Total					
	886.1	15.9	32.1	<0.0000	47.3
Arm flexed and tensed girth	−22.8				
Subscapular skinfold	5.4				
Tibiale mediale length	5.9				

represented by the acromial height and the arm length [11]. In our study, stature characterized only 1.9% (NS) and 3.8% (p < 0.05) of the total variance in boys and girls, respectively, while body weight characterized 18.4 and 17.4% in boys and girls, respectively. The best predictor of body resistance was stature and weight combined (27.1 and 20.7%, respectively) slightly higher than BMI (25.5 and 20.2%, respectively).

Houtkooper et al. [12] using S^2/R to predict FFM, concluded that more information is needed regarding the size and shape of the conductor than that provided by stature in children aged 10–14 years. Roche and Guo [13] derived an equation to predict FFM in 7- to 25-year-old males. They included S^2/R, weight, two skinfolds, and arm muscle circumference indices as independent variables to the equation. Therefore, there is an urgent need to use additional anthropometric measures rather than stature also to present new equations for calculation of body composition in children.

In a study of young adults (18–30 years of age) using weight, upper arm and calf circumferences, and seven skinfold thicknesses it was found that about 70% of the variance in resistance could be accounted for by a small set of anthropometric variables such as arm and calf circumferences [14]. Chumlea et al. [15] demonstrated that the use of shoulder height and arm length rather than stature as a measure of length of the conductor marginally improved the accuracy of the predictor. To date, such associations in young children have not been published.

Results of the current study indicated that best predictors on body resistance were girth parameters which characterized about 30–50% of total variance in prepubertal children. Surprisingly, not only small diameter limb girths, but gluteal in boys and waist in girls were added to the prediction model. Girth ratios such as waist/hip and waist/thigh have been used by most investigators as a measure of fat distribution with variable results. In the present study, correlations between body resistance and waist/thigh ratio were only moderate but significant in boys and girls. Organ et al. [16] showed that both indexes correlated significantly with the impedance index in adults. Probably, the waist/thigh girth ratio is more important because this ratio contains the girth of the lower limb in which resistance is relatively high.

As in adults [2, 10], length parameters only slightly influenced body resistance in children (tables 2–4). This is surprising as the body resistance depends on the conductor length. Potentially, the very small girths of the upper and lower body in children is a higher predictor than the length of the limbs. The influence of skinfold thicknesses to the body resistance is low, characterizing less than 10% of the total variance (tables 3,4). The sum of skinfolds characterized 7.2% of body resistance in girls and 2.4% in boys. This is due to the fact that body fat is a very bad electric conductor [1, 2, 10].

In conclusion, the traditional use of body stature as a single anthropometric measure used in the presentation of equations for body composition measurement is not acceptable. It is important to add girth parameters to stature in the prediction of body composition in preadolescent children.

Acknowledgements

We express thanks to professors Albrecht Claessens and Han Kemper for their comments and suggestions.

References

1   Lukaski HC: Assessment of body composition using tetrapolar bioelectrical impedance analysis; in Whitehead RG, Prentice A (eds): New Techniques in Nutritional Research. San Diego: Academic Press 1991, pp 303–315.

2   Kushner RF: Bioelectrical impedance analysis: A review of principles and applications. J Am Coll Nutr 1992;11:199–209.

3   Deurenberg P: Multi-frequency impedance as a measure of body water compartments; in Davies PSW, Cole TJ (eds): Body Composition Techniques in Health and Disease. London, Cambridge University Press, 1995, pp 45–56.

4   Fuller NJ, Elia M: Potential use of bioelectric impedance of the 'whole body' and of body segments for the assessment of body composition: Comparison with densitometry. Eur J Clin Nutr 1989;43: 779–791.

5   Chumlea WC, Baumgartner RN, Roche AF: Specific resistivity used to estimate fat free mass from segmental body measures of bioelectric impedance. Am J Clin Nutr 1988;48:7–15.

6   Fomon SJ, Haschke F, Ziegler EE, Nelson SE: Body composition of reference male children from birth to 10 years. Am J Clin Nutr 1982;35:1169–1175.

7   Hewitt MJ, Going SB, Williams DP, Lohmann TG: Hydration of fat-free body in children and adults: Implications for body composition assessment. Am J Physiol 1993;265:E88.

8   Tanner JM: Growth at Adolescence, ed 2. Oxford, Blackwell Scientific Publications, 1962

9   Norton KI, Whittingham N, Carter JEL, Kerr D, Gore C, Marfell-Jones MJ: Measurement techniques in anthropometry; in Norton KI, Olds TS (eds): Anthropometrica. Sydney, UNSW Press, 1996, pp 25–75.

10 Baumgartner RN, Chumlea WC, Roche AF: Bioelectric impedance for body composition. Exerc Sci Rev 1990;18:193–224.

11 Grieve C, Henneberg M: Statistical significance of body impedance measurements in estimating body composition. Homo 1998;49:1–12.

12 Houtkooper LB, Lohman TG, Going SB, Hall MC, Harrison GG: Validity of whole-body bioelectrical impedance analysis for body composition assessment in children. Med Sci Sports Exerc 1987; 19:S39.

13 Roche AF, Guo S: Biased estimation of fat-free mass. Proc Biopharmaceutical Section. Ann Meet Am Statistical Assoc, New Orleans, 1988, pp 188–191.

14 Baumgartner RN, Chumlea WC, Roche AF: Associations between bioelectrical impedance and anthropometric variables. Hum Biol 1987;59:235–244.

15 Chumlea WC, Baumgartner RN, Roche AF: The use of specific resistivity to estimate fat-free mass from segmental body measures of bioelectric impedance. Am J Clin Nutr 1988;48:7–15.

16 Organ LW, Bradham GB, Gore DT, Delozier SL: Segmental bioelectrical impedance analysis: Theory and application for a new technique. J Appl Physiol 1994;77:98–112.

Prof. Toivo Jürimäe, PhD, University of Tartu, 18 Ülikooli Street, 51014 Tartu (Estonia)
Tel. +372 7 375 372, Fax +372 7 375 373, E-Mail toivoj@ut.ee

Jürimäe T, Hills AP (eds): Body Composition Assessment in Children and Adolescents.
Med Sport Sci. Basel, Karger, 2001, vol 44, pp 71–84

....

Relationships between Anthropometric Parameters and Sexual Maturation in 12- to 15-Year-Old Estonian Girls

Gudrun Veldre[a], *Toivo Jürimäe*[b], *Helje Kaarma*[c]

[a] Institute of Zoology and Hydrobiology, Centre for Physical Anthropology
[b] Institute of Sport Pedagogy, and
[c] Centre for Physical Anthropology, University of Tartu, Estonia

The most variable component of human body composition, fat tissue, ranges from approximately 5% to over 50% of body mass [1]. There has been increasing scientific interest in fat mass largely because of its relationship to health status [2–5]. However, there are still some difficulties in the accurate estimation of body fat, particularly in children [6–8].

It is evident that the prediction of fat percentage by skinfolds depends on a range of factors including sex, ethnicity, age and the site of the measured skinfold [7, 9, 10]. Many studies have recommended that an increase in the number of measurement sites reduces errors and corrects possible differences in fat distribution between individuals within the same age and sex group [4, 11]. Some authors [12, 13] have shown that the relationship between skinfold thickness and body fat percentage depends on body size. Furthermore, the dimensions of the body should also be considered in the prediction equations. Studies of body composition based on skinfold measurements show that the sum of skinfolds is more indicative of subcutaneous fat than single skinfolds [14].

A small number of investigations have addressed the relationships between skinfold thicknesses and other anthropometric variables and sexual maturity characteristics in children [10, 15] and young athletes [16, 17]. Generally, investigations on the relationship between biological maturation and anthropometric characteristics of a given population use two different methodologies: correlation analysis or contrasting of maturity groups [17, 18]. At all age levels between 6 and 16 years, more mature girls are characterised by larger body dimensions and subcutaneous adipose tissue thicknesses than slower maturing girls but the correlations between these variables and the timing of maturation were relatively low, even in girls [17, 19]. Later maturation was generally observed for girls of a more linear build and lower body mass for stature [20, 21]. Differences between contrasting maturity groups increase until puberty. While the general sequence of pubertal events is remarkably constant, there is considerable variability in detail including in the time spent in any given stage of puberty [22]. The substantial variability in maturational status and morphological characteristics (including skinfolds) may be the major cause of the limited number of studies to consider the relationship between body composition change and indicators of pubertal maturation [23].

The aim of this study was to investigate changes in the main anthropometric parameters (skinfolds, girths, lengths, and ratios between breadth and length) at the different stages of maturation in girls.

Materials and Methods

In total, 394 12- to 15-year-old Estonian children and adolescents participated in this investigation. All subjects were residents of the city of Tartu (approximately 100,000 inhabitants), Estonia, and all were of Estonian origin. The children had no known chronic diseases and none of them were heavily involved in any sports as assessed using a self-reported questionnaire. However, subjects participated in two compulsory physical education lessons per week. Parents and children consented to voluntary testing. The study was approved by the Medical Ethics Committee of the University of Tartu.

Measurements were performed in the morning at school after emptying the bladder. All children had a light traditional breakfast and did not exercise before the testing session. Stature was measured using a Martin metal anthropometer in cm (± 0.1 cm) and body mass with medical scales in kg (± 0.05 kg) and BMI (kg/m^2) was calculated. In total, nine skinfolds (triceps, subscapular, biceps, iliac crest, supraspinale, abdominal, front thigh, medial calf, mid-axilla) were measured. In addition, 13 girths (head, neck, arm relaxed, arm flexed and tensed, forearm, wrist, chest, waist, gluteal, thigh, mid trochanter-tibiale laterale, calf, ankle), eight lengths (acromiale-radiale, radiale-stylion, midstylion-dactylion, iliospinale-box height, trochanterion-box height, trochanterion-tibiale-laterale, tibiale-laterale to floor, tibiale mediale-sphyrion tibiale) were recorded. Further, eight breadths/lengths (biacromial, biiliocristal, foot length, sitting height, transverse chest, A-P chest, humerus, femur) were measured. The series of anthropometric measurements were taken by a trained anthropometrist who had previously shown test-retest reliability of $r > 0.90$. The CENTURION KIT instrumentation was used (Rosscraft, Surrey, BC, Canada) for girth, length and breadth/length measurements. The skinfold thicknesses were measured using Holtain (Crymmych, UK) skinfold calipers. Calibration of all equipment was conducted prior to and at regular intervals during the data collection period. The nine measures of skinfold thicknesses were summed. All anthropometric variables were measured according to the protocol recommended by the International Society for Advancement of Kinanthropometry [24].

Pubertal status of the subjects was measured using the Tanner [20] stages. The self-assessment technique was used and both pubic hair (PH1, PH2, PH3, PH4, PH5) and breast (MA1, MA2, MA3, MA4, MA5) development were assessed. Girls were asked about the exact age and onset of menarche.

Standard statistical methods were used to calculate mean ($\bar{X}$) and standard deviation ($\pm$SD). Statistical comparisons of anthropometric parameters between different chronological ages and different pubertal stages of participants were made using two-way ANOVAs. Significance was set at $p \leq 0.05$.

Results

The mean age at menarche for girls (n = 190) was 12.96 $\pm$ 0.89 years. The earliest age at which menarche occurred was 10.44 years and the maximal age at menarche was 14.75 years. Mean anthropometric parameters selected by chronological age are presented in table 1. During puberty, especially at the beginning of puberty, the increase in body mass and BMI was not as intense as at the age of 14 and 15. However, body stature increased significantly, especially between 13 and 14 years, although the increase was already statistically significant between 12 and 13 years.

Most of the skinfold thicknesses were significantly greater at the age of 15 compared with the age of 12 (table 1). Surprisingly, the sum of skinfolds did not increase significantly across these years. Compared with skinfolds, most girths increased significantly between 12 and 14 years of age. For some girths, there were already significant differences from the age of 13 to 14 (neck, gluteal, thigh (1 cm gluteal)). The differences were only significant between the age of 12 and 15 for wrist and chest girth.

Limb length changes were similar to most girths although for some of them (iliospinale height, tibiale mediale-sphyrion tibiale) the changes were statistically significant between the age of 12 and 13. Changes in breadths/lengths were similar to length parameters and for some of these (biacromial length and A-P chest depth) changes were significant between the ages of 12 and 13. For other length parameters (biiliocristal height, sitting height, transverse chest), significant changes occurred between the age of 13 and 14 years. Thus the significant changes were between the age of 12 and 14 for most of breadths/lengths (table 1).

Body stature was highly dependent on the stage of biological maturation (table 2). The stature spurt was especially high (p < 0.05) between the first stages (MA1-MA2, MA2-MA3 or PH1-PH2, PH2-PH3). Body mass also increased substantially at this time but the first differences were significant only between stages 2 and 3.

The skinfold thicknesses increased significantly from the MA stages 1 to 3 and PH stages 1 to 4 (table 2). Highest statistical differences occurred between

Table 1. Mean ($\bar{X} \pm SD$) physical and anthropometric characteristics selected by chronological age in girls

Variable	12 years old (n = 84)	13 years old (n = 110)	14 years old (n = 105)	15 years old (n = 97)
Mass, kg	42.86 ± 9.12	46.33 ± 9.38	50.93 ± 9.12*	53.83 ± 8.01*
Height, cm	154.53 ± 8.01	157.87 ± 7.04*	162.29 ± 6.52*	164.81 ± 5.43*
BMI, kg/m²	17.81 ± 2.59	18.45 ± 2.70	19.26 ± 2.80*	19.75 ± 2.36*
Skinfolds, mm				
Triceps	10.48 ± 3.80	10.87 ± 3.96	12.04 ± 4.47	13.24 ± 4.11*
Subscapular	7.53 ± 3.77	8.06 ± 3.49	9.29 ± 4.06	10.20 ± 5.09*
Biceps	6.23 ± 2.49	6.56 ± 3.08	6.79 ± 3.11	7.33 ± 2.74
Iliac crest	9.91 ± 5.11	11.05 ± 6.44	12.20 ± 5.87	14.27 ± 6.83*
Supraspinale	6.48 ± 3.58	7.04 ± 3.96	7.88 ± 4.02	8.94 ± 5.19*
Abdominal	11.19 ± 6.68	11.62 ± 6.77	13.26 ± 6.88	15.37 ± 7.62*
Front thigh	20.46 ± 8.32	21.25 ± 9.23	22.23 ± 9.04	26.96 ± 9.75*
Medial calf	12.41 ± 5.11	12.61 ± 5.38	13.50 ± 4.92	14.54 ± 4.67
Mid-axilla	7.04 ± 4.62	7.00 ± 3.94	7.50 ± 3.19	8.53 ± 5.06
Sum of skinfolds	91.37 ± 39.59	96.05 ± 42.81	104.69 ± 40.42	119.90 ± 45.25
Girths, cm				
Head	54.25 ± 1.56	54.67 ± 1.77	55.30 ± 1.58*	55.45 ± 1.50*
Neck	29.49 ± 1.61	29.99 ± 1.67	30.91 ± 1.63*	31.60 ± 1.54*
Arm (relaxed)	22.40 ± 2.81	23.08 ± 2.79	24.06 ± 2.91*	24.70 ± 2.35*
Arm (flexed and tensed)	23.42 ± 2.67	24.19 ± 2.66	25.23 ± 2.89*	25.72 ± 2.27*
Forearm (maximum)	21.59 ± 1.93	22.14 ± 1.64	22.83 ± 1.74*	23.11 ± 1.41*
Wrist (distal styloids)	14.57 ± 0.92	14.71 ± 0.93	15.01 ± 0.97	15.15 ± 0.77*
Chest (mesosternale)	77.05 ± 6.35	77.34 ± 6.13	80.00 ± 5.87	82.08 ± 5.63*
Waist (minimum)	62.38 ± 5.87	63.43 ± 5.68	65.27 ± 5.53*	66.86 ± 5.65*
Gluteal (hips)	81.73 ± 7.78	84.84 ± 7.64	89.30 ± 7.45*	91.47 ± 5.28*
Thigh (1 cm gluteal)	48.03 ± 5.38	49.76 ± 5.44	52.22 ± 5.53*	53.27 ± 4.05*
Thigh (medial)	42.84 ± 4.56	44.29 ± 4.80	46.01 ± 4.87*	46.98 ± 3.42*
Calf (maximum)	31.52 ± 2.94	32.32 ± 2.91	33.52 ± 2.87*	34.25 ± 2.25*
Ankle (minimum)	21.15 ± 1.53	21.43 ± 1.54	21.93 ± 1.73*	22.21 ± 1.17*
Lengths, cm				
Acromiale-radiale	28.10 ± 1.95	28.87 ± 1.83	29.64 ± 1.60*	30.28 ± 1.56*
Radiale-stylion	23.10 ± 1.45	23.82 ± 1.49	24.18 ± 1.25*	24.51 ± 1.13*
Midstylion-dactylion	16.75 ± 1.09	17.04 ± 0.79	17.39 ± 0.87*	17.62 ± 0.74*
Iliospinale ht	87.80 ± 5.59	90.29 ± 4.80*	92.00 ± 3.87*	93.06 ± 4.31*
Trochanterion ht	82.12 ± 4.97	83.62 ± 4.77	85.20 ± 3.86*	87.09 ± 4.16*
Trochanterion-tibiale laterale	40.94 ± 2.70	41.21 ± 2.77	42.00 ± 2.53	43.79 ± 1.93*
Tibiale laterale to floor	40.80 ± 2.55	41.85 ± 2.68	42.31 ± 2.06*	42.58 ± 2.17*
Tibiale mediale-sphy.tibiale	34.82 ± 2.30	36.34 ± 2.77*	37.10 ± 2.20*	36.78 ± 2.05*
Breadths/Lengths, cm				
Biacromial	32.27 ± 2.01	33.26 ± 1.70*	33.94 ± 1.78*	34.26 ± 1.91*
Biiliocristal	24.33 ± 1.80	25.09 ± 1.76	26.23 ± 1.72*	26.70 ± 1.61*
Foot length	23.90 ± 1.31	24.18 ± 1.02	24.34 ± 1.13	24.62 ± 0.98*
Sitting height	80.00 ± 3.98	81.53 ± 4.09	84.71 ± 3.83*	86.32 ± 2.77*
Transverse chest	22.80 ± 1.89	23.12 ± 1.53	24.05 ± 1.48*	24.48 ± 1.64*
A-P chest depth	15.99 ± 1.44	16.74 ± 1.58*	16.93 ± 1.64*	17.29 ± 1.39*
Humerus	5.85 ± 0.34	5.87 ± 0.33	5.98 ± 0.32	6.01 ± 0.28*
Femur	8.38 ± 0.46	8.41 ± 0.45	8.54 ± 0.46	8.57 ± 0.41

* Statistically significant (p < 0.05) difference with age 12.

Table 2. Mean ($\bar{X} \pm SD$) skinfold thicknesses selected by breast development (MA) and pubic hair (PH) development stage

Variable	MA 1 (n=14)	MA 2 (n=70)	MA3 (n=169)	MA 4 (n=122)	MA 5 (n=19)
Chronological age	12.34±0.47	12.75±0.76	13.41±0.92*	14.24±0.88*	14.63±0.66*
Height, cm	146.56±8.14	153.75±7.02*	160.29±6.45*	163.89±5.40*	165.07±8.29*
Mass, kg	33.45±3.98	40.37±6.80	48.62±8.38 *	53.49±8.01*	59.16±0.51*
BMI, kg/m²	15.57±1.24	17.04±2.09	18.84±2.44*	19.87±2.48*	21.58±3.33*
Skinfold, mm					
Triceps	8.12±2.02	9.72±3.44	11.56±3.83*	12.68±3.93*	16.38±6.72*
Subscapular	5.21±0.66	7.03±3.88	8.46±3.38	10.00±4.52*	13.29±6.15*
Biceps	4.34±1.21	5.79±2.80	6.59±2.64	7.33±2.71*	9.62±4.46*
Iliac crest	5.47±1.66	8.97±5.00	11.32±5.47*	14.10±6.37*	18.75±8.25*
Supraspinale	3.89±1.00	5.69±2.92	7.48±4.01*	8.57±4.25*	12.56±6.71*
Abdominal	5.91±2.86	9.59±5.95	12.92±6.93*	14.52±6.58*	19.54±9.61*
Front thigh	13.47±4.12	19.01±8.60	22.75±8.93*	24.71±9.26*	30.75±10.64*
Medial calf	8.18±2.67	11.29±4.79	13.37±5.11*	14.33±4.42*	16.94±6.30*
Mid-axilla	4.68±1.27	6.13±3.81	7.38±3.97	8.25±4.01	11.29±7.08*
Sum of skinfolds	59.28±13.08	83.22±37.71	101.69±39.45*	114.85±41.00*	149.13±57.74*

	PH 1 (n=33)	PH 2 (n=74)	PH 3 (n=105)	PH 4 (n=156)	PH 5 (n=26)
Chronological age	12.49±0.79	12.90±0.78	13.30±0.86*	14.12±0.91*	14.59±0.69*
Height, cm	149.81±8.47	154.66±6.75*	159.96±5.93*	163.79±5.78*	165.33±5.04*
Mass, kg	37.68±8.36	42.39±7.19	48.38±8.10*	52.83±8.79*	56.38±8.79*
BMI, kg/m²	16.62±2.31	17.67±2.19	18.83±2.39*	19.65±2.79*	20.43±2.52*
Skinfold, mm					
Triceps	9.93±3.90	10.17±3.01	11.37±3.94	12.50±4.37*	14.65±5.20*
Subscapular	6.93±4.46	7.19±3.05	8.60±4.01	9.69±4.28*	11.28±5.18*
Biceps	5.75±2.77	5.99±2.63	6.78±2.96	7.12±2.95	7.75±2.77
Iliac crest	8.73±4.92	9.42±5.23	11.56±5.62	13.30±6.64*	16.16±6.83*
Supraspinale	5.88±3.84	5.95±2.95	7.39±3.83	8.40±4.51*	10.75±5.95*
Abdominal	9.76±6.72	9.87±5.66	12.79±6.70	14.29±7.15*	17.49±8.74*
Front thigh	17.90±7.99	20.36±8.39	22.04±8.85	24.50±9.80*	28.00±9.70*
Medial calf	10.41±4.61	12.05±4.71	13.00±5.03	14.33±5.12*	15.30±4.52*
Mid-axilla	6.36±4.24	5.99±3.05	7.31±3.67	8.20±4.39	10.10±6.31*
Sum of skinfolds	81.66±39.41	86.98±35.07	100.62±40.22	112.60±44.21*	131.50±47.76*

* Statistically significant (p<0.05) difference with stage 1.

stages MA2 and MA3 in some skinfolds (triceps, supraspinale and abdominal). Subscapular and iliac crest skinfolds had most pronounced statistically significant changes between the stages MA3 and MA4. The rate of increase was lowest between stages MA3 and MA4 for all measured limb skinfolds and for supraspinale, abdominal and mid-axilla skinfolds. The triceps, subscapular, biceps and supraspinale skinfold thicknesses increased significantly from stage MA4 to MA5. Mid-axilla skinfold differed from other skinfolds at this point and increase at this site was statistically significant only between MA and PH stages 1 and 5.

The biggest differences for stages by MA and PH were in biceps skinfold, which increased significantly with ascending MA stages but not with gain of PH stages (table 2). There were two increases: between MA1-MA2 and then between MA4-MA5 subgroups for some skinfolds (medial calf and front thigh) ($p < 0.05$).

Changes in the girth parameters at the period of maturation are presented in table 3. Most of the measured girths increased significantly at the beginning of sexual maturation. There were significant differences between MA and PH stages 1 and 3 (and also between MA2-MA3). Significant changes occurred first between stages MA1 and MA2, but between PH2 and PH3 for forearm, chest (mesosternale) and gluteal girths.

The length parameters also increased significantly during different stages of puberty (table 4). The significant differences were already seen between stages MA1 and MA2 for one group of lengths (radiale-stylion, iliospinale height, trochanterion height, tibiale mediale-sphyrion tibiale). This coincides with a rapid increased in total body stature (table 2). The first significant changes were observed between stages MA2 and MA3 for the second part of lengths (acromiale-radiale, midstylion dactylion, trochanterion-tibiale laterale, tibiale laterale to floor). Significant differences in lengths by PH stages occurred mostly between stages PH2-PH3, with the exception of the acromiale-radiale length that significantly changes already between PH1 and PH2, which was different from means of MA stages.

Significant differences occurred between stages MA2-MA3 on all breadths/lengths parameters (table 5) as was the case on body mass. For some breadths/lengths (biacromial breadths, bicristal breadths, sitting height, transverse chest) significant differences were also found between MA3 and MA4. Significant changes in some breadths also began with minor PH stages in comparison with MA stages. Significant changes in biacromial breadth, sitting height and A-P chest depth existed between PH stages 1 and 2 and between MA stages 2 and 3.

Most anthropometric variables in 12- to 15-year-old girls increased with advancing age and maturity signs (tables 1–5). The means of subgroups formed

Table 3. Mean ($\bar{X} \pm$ SD) girths selected by breast development (MA) and pubic hair (PH) development stage

Variable	MA 1 (n = 14)	MA 2 (n = 70)	MA3 (n = 169)	MA 4 (n = 122)	MA 5 (n = 19)
Girths, cm					
Head	53.06 ± 1.34	53.83 ± 1.77	54.90 ± 1.47*	55.71 ± 1.41*	55.83 ± 1.37*
Neck	28.05 ± 1.22	29.14 ± 1.53	30.39 ± 1.47*	31.52 ± 1.50*	32.19 ± 1.76*
Arm (relaxed)	19.83 ± 1.70	21.58 ± 2.18	23.61 ± 2.59*	24.74 ± 2.45*	26.25 ± 3.35*
Arm (flexed and tensed)	20.99 ± 1.59	22.66 ± 2.09	24.65 ± 2.43*	25.86 ± 2.36*	27.44 ± 3.37*
Forearm (maximum)	19.52 ± 2.05	21.17 ± 1.35*	22.50 ± 1.52*	23.20 ± 1.45*	23.86 ± 1.89*
Wrist (distal styloids)	13.67 ± 0.73	14.27 ± 0.74	14.90 ± 0.84*	15.20 ± 0.85*	15.47 ± 1.05*
Chest (mesosternale)	66.99 ± 3.57	74.45 ± 5.50*	78.42 ± 5.73*	81.59 ± 5.40*	85.32 ± 7.45*
Waist (minimum)	57.16 ± 3.34	61.18 ± 4.60	64.46 ± 5.22*	66.58 ± 5.58*	69.98 ± 7.81*
Gluteal (hips)	73.51 ± 3.79	79.82 ± 6.05*	87.02 ± 6.71*	91.27 ± 5.80*	95.58 ± 7.28*
Thigh (1 cm gluteal)	42.54 ± 2.97	46.42 ± 4.11	51.02 ± 4.88*	53.30 ± 4.33*	56.73 ± 5.98*
Thigh (medial)	38.34 ± 2.50	41.40 ± 3.46	45.29 ± 4.36*	47.02 ± 3.81*	49.71 ± 4.80*
Calf (maximum)	28.90 ± 1.87	30.63 ± 2.11	32.95 ± 2.70*	34.29 ± 2.40*	35.63 ± 2.93*
Ankle (minimum)	19.74 ± 1.29	20.75 ± 1.24	21.77 ± 1.52*	22.25 ± 1.41*	22.37 ± 1.43*

	PH 1 (n = 33)	PH 2 (n = 74)	PH 3 (n = 105)	PH 4 (n = 156)	PH 5 (n = 26)
Girths, cm					
Head	53.42 ± 1.72	54.19 ± 1.76	54.90 ± 1.49*	55.57 ± 1.40*	55.38 ± 1.54*
Neck	28.66 ± 1.53	29.53 ± 1.61	30.36 ± 1.61*	31.26 ± 1.51*	31.92 ± 1.48*
Arm (relaxed)	21.26 ± 2.70	22.11 ± 2.24	23.63 ± 2.69*	24.46 ± 2.69*	25.43 ± 2.61*
Arm (flexed and tensed)	22.24 ± 2.52	23.17 ± 2.14	24.78 ± 2.56*	25.52 ± 2.56*	26.54 ± 2.76*
Forearm (maximum)	20.53 ± 2.05	21.46 ± 1.34	22.55 ± 1.55*	23.07 ± 1.56*	23.45 ± 1.58*
Wrist (distal styloids)	14.00 ± 0.92	14.46 ± 0.81	14.89 ± 0.85*	15.13 ± 0.86*	15.44 ± 0.83*
Chest (mesosternale)	75.45 ± 7.14	75.63 ± 5.18	78.31 ± 5.73	81.03 ± 6.00*	83.55 ± 6.19*
Waist (minimum)	59.64 ± 5.08	61.96 ± 4.84	64.42 ± 5.03*	66.31 ± 5.95*	67.95 ± 6.14*
Gluteal (hips)	77.57 ± 7.96	81.69 ± 6.38	86.79 ± 6.35*	90.50 ± 6.77*	93.54 ± 5.55*
Thigh (1 cm gluteal)	45.09 ± 5.01	47.88 ± 4.42	50.76 ± 4.74*	52.96 ± 5.15*	54.87 ± 3.97*
Thigh (medial)	40.10 ± 3.98	42.71 ± 3.93	45.04 ± 4.28*	46.79 ± 4.38*	48.36 ± 3.20*
Calf (maximum)	29.87 ± 2.51	31.39 ± 2.52	32.86 ± 2.64*	34.07 ± 2.63*	34.79 ± 2.47*
Ankle (minimum)	20.15 ± 1.49	21.02 ± 1.42	21.71 ± 1.35*	22.22 ± 1.46*	22.39 ± 1.38

* Statistically significant ($p < 0.05$) difference with stage 1.
* The mean chronological age, body height and mass and BMI of different groups is presented in table 2.

Table 4. Mean ($\bar{X} \pm SD$) lengths selected by breast development (MA) and pubic hair (PH) development stage

Variable	MA 1 (n = 14)	MA 2 (n = 70)	MA3 (n = 169)	MA 4 (n = 122)	MA 5 (n = 19)
Lengths, cm					
Acromiale-radiale	26.47 ± 1.92	27.92 ± 1.97	29.33 ± 1.55*	30.10 ± 1.61*	30.06 ± 1.81*
Radiale-stylion	21.73 ± 1.30	23.07 ± 1.36*	24.02 ± 1.31*	24.47 ± 1.16*	24.39 ± 1.40*
Midstylion-dactylion	15.93 ± 1.10	16.61 ± 0.91	17.27 ± 0.83*	17.56 ± 0.76*	17.58 ± 0.86*
Iliospinale ht	83.36 ± 6.01	87.86 ± 5.30*	91.32 ± 4.23*	92.70 ± 4.08*	91.93 ± 5.36*
Trochanterion ht	77.84 ± 4.83	81.74 ± 4.69*	84.84 ± 4.49*	86.36 ± 3.79*	85.73 ± 4.52*
Trochanterion-tibiale laterale	38.97 ± 2.62	40.37 ± 2.50	42.06 ± 2.72*	43.04 ± 2.24*	42.74 ± 2.26*
Tibiale laterale to floor	38.96 ± 3.40	40.74 ± 2.21	42.09 ± 2.34*	42.71 ± 2.17*	41.98 ± 2.27*
Tibiale mediale-sphy.tibiale	32.78 ± 2.68	35.35 ± 2.38*	36.59 ± 2.32*	36.80 ± 2.22*	36.97 ± 3.04*

	PH 1 (n = 33)	PH 2 (n = 74)	PH 3 (n = 105)	PH 4 (n = 156)	PH 5 (n = 26)
Lengths, cm					
Acromiale-radiale	26.81 ± 2.18	28.30 ± 1.67*	29.40 ± 1.51*	29.95 ± 1.63*	30.25 ± 1.39*
Radiale-stylion	22.53 ± 1.65	23.20 ± 1.34	24.08 ± 1.33*	24.37 ± 1.16*	24.47 ± 1.28*
Midstylion-dactylion	16.29 ± 1.21	16.76 ± 0.90	17.24 ± 0.83*	17.55 ± 0.74*	17.49 ± 0.60*
Iliospinale ht	85.49 ± 5.89	88.04 ± 4.67	91.36 ± 4.27*	92.80 ± 4.11*	92.30 ± 4.04*
Trochanterion ht	79.53 ± 4.79	81.98 ± 4.25	84.88 ± 4.45*	86.28 ± 4.12*	86.54 ± 3.41*
Trochanterion-tibiale laterale	39.64 ± 2.88	40.56 ± 2.64	41.97 ± 2.40*	42.90 ± 2.48*	43.59 ± 1.65*
Tibiale laterale to floor	39.82 ± 2.90	40.86 ± 2.15	42.30 ± 2.46*	42.54 ± 2.18*	42.41 ± 1.89*
Tibiale mediale-sphy.tibiale	34.08 ± 2.83	35.23 ± 2.50	36.61 ± 2.28*	37.01 ± 2.25*	36.93 ± 1.56*

* Statistically significant ($p < 0.05$) difference with stage 1.
* The mean chronological age, body height and mass and BMI of different groups is presented in table 2.

according to the secondary sexual characteristics had greater differences among themselves than means of subgroups made by chronological age. The data demonstrated that the differences between girls with different chronological age (12–15) were smaller (table 1) than the differences between the girls with different breast (MA1-MA5) or pubic hair (PH1-PH5) development (tables 2–5). All data showed that the largest increments were between developmental stages 1 and 2 (by breast development between MA1 to MA2; by pubic hair between PH1 to PH2) for one part of the variables.

Table 5. Mean ($\bar{X} \pm$ SD) breadths/lengths selected by breast development (MA) and pubic hair (PH) development stage

Variable	MA 1 (n = 14)	MA 2 (n = 70)	MA3 (n = 169)	MA 4 (n = 122)	MA 5 (n = 19)
Breadths/lengths, cm					
Biacromial	30.74 ± 2.00	32.07 ± 1.68	33.54 ± 1.66*	34.29 ± 1.79*	34.84 ± 2.01*
Biiliocristal	22.93 ± 1.36	24.04 ± 1.69	25.60 ± 1.63*	26.57 ± 1.56*	27.45 ± 1.94*
Foot length	23.12 ± 1.32	23.78 ± 1.09	24.39 ± 1.12*	24.55 ± 1.00*	24.25 ± 0.99
Sitting height	76.05 ± 3.25	79.04 ± 3.50	83.13 ± 3.56*	85.85 ± 2.95*	87.43 ± 4.82*
Transverse chest	21.36 ± 1.33	22.44 ± 1.45	23.63 ± 1.54*	24.33 ± 1.52*	25.22 ± 2.14*
A-P chest depth	14.60 ± 1.01	15.79 ± 1.46	16.82 ± 1.43*	17.33 ± 1.40*	17.56 ± 1.90*
Humerus	5.51 ± 0.30	5.78 ± 0.28	5.94 ± 0.32*	6.03 ± 0.29*	6.02 ± 0.29*
Femur	8.00 ± 0.33	8.26 ± 0.37	8.49 ± 0.44*	8.60 ± 0.44*	8.70 ± 0.45*

	PH 1 (n = 33)	PH 2 (n = 74)	PH 3 (n = 105)	PH 4 (n = 156)	PH 5 (n = 26)
Breadths/lengths, cm					
Biacromial	31.44 ± 2.12	32.58 ± 1.80*	33.33 ± 1.63*	34.21 ± 1.70*	34.74 ± 2.05*
Biiliocristal	23.42 ± 1.89	24.42 ± 1.69	25.63 ± 1.54*	26.39 ± 1.63*	27.20 ± 1.75*
Foot length	23.45 ± 1.54	23.94 ± 1.00	24.32 ± 1.05*	24.58 ± 1.05*	24.31 ± 0.94
Sitting height	77.71 ± 4.08	79.96 ± 3.84*	82.70 ± 3.27*	85.58 ± 3.28*	87.19 ± 3.00*
Transverse chest	22.00 ± 1.84	22.79 ± 1.44	23.52 ± 1.40*	24.19 ± 1.63*	25.17 ± 1.82*
A-P chest depth	15.13 ± 1.48	16.19 ± 1.35*	16.82 ± 1.52*	17.24 ± 1.46*	17.22 ± 1.56*
Humerus	5.70 ± 0.35	5.82 ± 0.29	5.94 ± 0.33*	6.01 ± 0.30*	5.98 ± 0.31*
Femur	8.19 ± 0.42	8.33 ± 0.40	8.49 ± 0.38*	8.56 ± 0.48*	8.72 ± 0.46*

* Statistically significant ($p < 0.05$) difference with stage 1.

* The mean chronological age, body height and mass and BMI of different groups is presented in table 2.

Discussion

Studies on growth and maturation have stressed that knowledge of the maturity status of the child, either from skeletal status or the development of secondary sex characteristics is important in the timing of pubescence and can allow better judgements of the normality of growth [19]. Though the details of the genetic regulation of the growth and maturation process are not perfectly clear, studies of parent-child relationships have suggested that the body build of parents was related to the rate of maturation of their offspring [19]. Other studies have demonstrated that there are some differences between persons growing at different rates even in the adult years. For example, final mean stature at an adult age has been reported to be bigger in the late than in the early maturers [25].

Longitudinal studies of girls have showed that the greatest change in breast development occurs 2 years prior, and for pubic hair development 1 year prior to menarche [18]. Peak height velocity occurs about 1.2–1.5 years before menarche [26]. To determine the age at peak height velocity assumes that (longitudinal) data are available for about 3-year periods before and after this event [19]. This leads to the serious need to use all available data, also data from cross-sectional studies to assess maturation status during the pubertal years.

The current anthropometric study in girls in the period of puberty showed that the differences between age groups were often less noteworthy than differences between parameters of groups formed by stages of sexual maturation (tables 1–5). The differences between early and late maturers of the same age also exceeded the differences between sexes [25]. Despite this, the means are counted differently for boys and girls.

It cannot be assumed that because a population is delayed in sexual maturation it will also be delayed in skeletal maturation. Generally, breast and pubic hair development is consistent with the development of skeletal maturation [2, 19, 27].

Girls in the present study experienced menarche at a similar age and range as reported by other authors [18, 19, 28, 29] for urban girls. This result compares with the age of menarche in European countries reported by Eveleth and Tanner [2]. However, it should be noted that the retrospective method used in this study identified an earlier menarche [2].

Similar to other investigations [18, 20], the current study demonstrated steady progression with chronological age in breast and pubic hair development. Age-related changes in body mass and stature was also significant, as was the case in a study of Canadian girls of the same age [18]. Our study revealed significant differences in mean body stature between 12- and 13-year-olds and also between the ages of 13 and 14. Body mass also changed significantly between the ages of 13 and 14. However, the mean statistics of variables by breast and pubic hair development stages gave another more particular indication of changes during this period of rapid change.

Tanner [28], breast stage 2 is reached on average at the age 8–13 years, breast stage 5 at age 12–18. PH2 occur after breast stage 2 by some 0.2 to 0.6 years in most populations [2]. The difference between PH2 and MA2 seems to be by difference of mean chronological age rather 0.2 years or even less than more in Estonian girls (table 2). The interval between PH1 and PH2 is on average a little shorter than from MA1 to MA2. PH2 comes on average later than MA2, but the mean age for PH3 stage outrun the mean chronological age for MA3. The mean chronological age was earlier for PH4 and PH5 than for MA4 and MA5, but these differences were not statistically significant.

Similar to longitudinal growth data [19] our data demonstrated that the biggest increase in body stature (between MA1and MA2) forestall the changes in body mass and then the increment of height in girls decreased steadily (table 2). The same tendency was seen for PH stages. Statistically significant changes in BMI by MA stages were concurrent to body mass changes (between MA2-MA3 and MA3-MA4). The differences in BMI between age groups were only obvious between age 12 and 14 (15).

Changes in skinfolds across the study period showed the biggest variations. Changes with chronological age were not statistically significant in some (biceps, medial calf and mid-axilla). This could be considered an expression of one well-known phenomenon of 'average' in cross-sectional studies that does not summarize but betrays the data [28], especially in the rapid growing years, because the mean depends on the proportion of children in different maturation stages in the given age group. The changes in mean values were only significant for all other skinfolds between the ages of 12 and 15, except for the front thigh which also increased significantly from 14 to 15 years. The biggest increments occurred in trunk skinfolds: iliac crest, supraspinale, abdominal and subscapular skinfolds. Observations suggested that the central-ization of body fat during adolescence is associated with increased deposition on the upper rather than lower trunk region [29]. Girls in the present study showed that during the period of rapid change there was not such a pronounced increase in subcutaneous body fat on the upper trunk as on the iliac-hypogas-tric region and on the back.

Our data showed that some skinfolds (triceps, supraspinale and abdom-inal) increased significantly at the same stage as body mass (between stages MA2 and MA3). Subscapular and iliac crest skinfolds, which Roche [19] recommends should be included in the assessment of nutritional status of women, have most pronounced and significant changes between stages MA3 and MA4. The triceps, subscapular, biceps and supraspinale skinfolds had a statistically significant increase from stage MA4 to MA5. This parallels the results of the investigation of Rico et al. [30] using dual-energy X-ray absorpti-ometry. This investigation revealed that girls rated as Tanner stages 4 and 5 had greater body fat content than girls who were in stages 1 and 2 ($p < 0.001$). Eveleth and Tanner [2] also reported that a considerable increase in body fat deposition occurred at the triceps and subscapular sites after puberty. This was also seen in the current study where the largest statistically significant increase in triceps and subscapular skinfolds was between MA4 and MA5 stages, though for the triceps skinfold, the first increase was between stages

MA2 and MA3. The data of the Fels Study [19] showed that triceps values for girls also increased prior to PHV but declined near this event except at the 90th percentile level, then increased later. Most studies have reported that the changes during adolescence are most commonly associated with the centralization of body fat [3, 29]. In addition to the substantial increases in trunk skinfolds, triceps and thigh skinfold thicknesses also increased. Differences between skinfolds from stage MA1 to MA5 were greater than two times the differences in skinfolds between age groups of 12- and 15-year-olds.

Although the sum of skinfolds did not change significantly from the age 12 to 15 by MA and PH stages, there were significant differences in the same period for most skinfolds (between MA2-MA3 and MA4-MA5 and PH1-PH4). This may be due to very high standard deviations.

Roche [19] has reported that pubescent changes occur earlier in the bones of the hand and foot than in the proximal bones of the limb. Our data using breast maturation stages confirm these observations. Changes in the distal parts of limbs (forearm length (radiale-stylion), and calf length (tibiale mediale-sphyrion. tibiale)) were similar to changes in height from MA1 to MA2. The biggest changes in length parameters in the age period studied were in the proximal parts of limbs (length of arm (acromiale-radiale) and thigh (trochanterion-tibiale radiale)) and occurred between stages MA2 and MA3.

Breadth/lengths changes suggested that changes in minor PH stage in comparison with corresponding MA stages were in variables that we can call as stockiness parameters (biacromial breadth, sitting height and A-P chest depth). There were statistically significant differences between subgroups PH1 and PH2 differently from most of other characteristics. It is possible that variables significantly different by PH and MA stages, which changed from minor PH stage than MA stage (previously mentioned breadth/lengths and arm length) are related to the bigger mesomorphy rate. Possibly the advanced pubic hair maturation is related with the mesomorphy component. Carter and Heath [14] did not exclude the possibility that there are two triggers associated with the onset of adolescent maturation and changes in somatotype. Possibly, the advanced maturation is related at the same time to both endomorphy (as in girls) or mesomorphy (as in boys) [14].

The biggest changes in girths were in the arm (relaxed), thigh and gluteal hips circumferences, in sites where the skinfold thicknesses increased considerably. Different from all other girth changes, the chest (mesosternale) girth was statistically significant between all MA stages.

In our opinion, it is reasonable to study cross-sectionally at the time of puberty the anthropometric variability not only by age groups but also by stages of sexual maturity because these differences could show more detail about changes in parameters.

Use of groups formed by stages of sexual maturation provides the possibility to study the genetically regulated shaping of body dimensions and fat patterning closely related with the process of maturation. As there is some evidence that fat patterning is more influenced by genetic control than relative fatness (percentage of fat) [8], the study of fat patterning changes in adolescence by maturational status provides an opportunity for a more comprehensive investigation of its determination and developmental growth.

Conclusion

In 12- to 15-year-old girls the most pronounced changes according to chronological age were in skinfold thicknesses and body girths and segmental lengths, then in breadths/lengths. The most substantial increase in subcutaneous body fat in girls was on the iliac-hypogastric region and on the back (subscapular skinfold). The analysis of data by sexual maturation subgroups showed a different consequence in relation to breast and pubic hair development stages.

References

1   Spady DW: Normal body composition of infants and children; in: Body Composition Measurements in Infants and Children. Report 98th Ross Conf, Columbus, 1989, vol 98, pp 67–75.
2   Eveleth PB, Tanner JM: Worldwide Variation in Human Growth, ed 2. Cambridge, Cambridge University Press, 1990.
3   Bouchard C: Heredity and Regional Fat Distribution During Growth; in Hernández M, Argente J (eds): Human Growth: Basic and Clinical Aspects. Proc Sixth Int Cong Auxology, Madrid, 1991. New York, Experta Medica, 1992, pp 227–232.
4   Deurenberg P: Methods for determining fat mass and fat distribution. Acta Paediatr Suppl 1992; 383:53–57.
5   Rolland-Cachera MF: Prediction of adult body composition from infant and child measurements; in Davies PSW, Cole TJ (eds): Body Composition Techniques in Health and Disease. Cambridge, Cambridge University Press, 1995, pp 100–145.
6   Davies PSW: Anthropometry and body composition; in Ulijaszek SJ, Mascie-Taylor CGN (eds): Cambridge Studies in Biological Anthropology 14: Anthropometry: The Individual and the Population. Cambridge, Cambridge University Press, 1994, pp 130–140.
7   Norgan NG: The assessment of the body composition of populations; in Davies PSW, Cole TJ (eds): Body Composition Techniques in Health and Disease. Cambridge, Cambridge University Press, 1995, pp 195–221.
8   Norgan NG: Body composition; in Ulijaszek SJ, Johnston FE, Preece MA (eds): The Cambridge Encyclopedia of Human Growth and Development. Cambridge, Cambridge University Press 1998, pp 212–215.
9   Pollock ML, Jackson AS: Research progression in validation of clinical methods of assessing body composition. Med Sci Sport Exerc 1984;16:606–613.
10 Baumgartner RN, Roche AF, Guo S, Lohman T, Boileau RA, Slaughter MH: Adipose tissue distribution: The stability of principal components by sex, ethnicity and maturation stage. Hum Biol 1986;58:719–735.

11 Martin AD, Ross WD, Drinkwater DT, Clarys JP: Prediction of body fat by skinfold caliper: Assumptions and cadaver evidence. Int J Obes 1985;9(suppl 1):31–39.

12 Himes JH, Roche AF: Subcutaneous fatness and stature: Relationship from infancy to adulthood. Hum Biol 1986;58:737–750.

13 Martin AD, Drinkwater DT: Variability in the measures of body fat: Assumptions or technique? Sport Med 1991;11:277–288.

14 Carter JEL, Heath BH: Somatotyping – Development and applications; in Lasker GW, Mascie-Taylor CGN, Roberts DF (eds): Cambridge Studies in Biological Anthropology 5. Cambridge, Cambridge University Press,1990.

15 Forbes GB: Body size and composition of perimenarcheal girls. Am J Dis Child 1992;146:63–66.

16 Malina RM, Bouchard C: Growth, Maturation, and Physical Activity. Champaign, Human Kinetics, 1991.

17 Beunen G: Biological maturation and physical performance; in Duquet W, Day JAP (eds): Kinanthropometry IV. E&FN Spon, 1993, pp 215–235.

18 Little NG, Day JAP, Steinke L: Relationship of physical performance to maturation in perimenarcheal girls. Am J Hum Biol 1997;9:163–171.

19 Roche AF: Growth, maturation, and body composition: The Fels Longitudinal Study 1929–1991; in Lasker GW, Mascie-Taylor CGN, Roberts DF, Foley RA (eds): Cambridge Studies in Biological Anthropology 9. Cambridge, Cambridge University Press, 1992, pp 120–156.

20 Tanner JM: Growth and Adolescence. Oxford, Blackwell Scientific, 1962.

21 Susanne C, Bodzsár EB: Patterns of secular change of growth and development; in Bodzsár EB, Susanne C (eds): Secular Growth Changes in Europe. Budapest, Eötvös University Press, 1998, pp 5–26.

22 Preece MA, Pan H, Ratcliffe SG: Auxological aspects of male and female puberty. Acta Paediatr 1992;81(suppl 383):11–13.

23 Malina RM: Menarche in athletes: A synthesis and hypothesis. Ann Hum Biol 1983;10:1–24.

24 Norton KI, Whittingham N, Carter JEL, Kerr D, Gore C, Marfell-Jones MJ: Measurement technique in anthropometry; in Norton KI, Olds TS (eds): Anthropometrica. Sydney, University of New South Wales Press, 1996, pp 25–75.

25 Prokopec M: Early and late maturers. Anthrop Közl 1982;26:13–24.

26 Ohsawa S, Cheng-Ye J, Kasai N: Age at menarche and comparison of the growth and performance of pre- and post-menarcheal girls in China. Am J Hum Biol 1997;9:205–212.

27 Malina RM: Physical activity and training for sport as factors affecting growth and maturation; in Ulijaszek SI, Johnston FE, Preece MA (eds): The Cambridge Encyclopedia of Human Growth and Development. Cambridge, Cambridge University Press, 1998, pp 216–219.

28 Tanner JM: Growth as a Mirror of Conditions of Society. Stockholm, Stockholm Institute of Education Press, 1990, pp 9–48.

29 Johnston, FE: Developmental aspects of fat patterning; in Hernández M, Argente J (eds) Human Growth: Basic and Clinical Aspects. Proc Sixth Int Congr Auxology, Madrid, 1991. New York, Experta Medica, 1992, pp 217–226.

30 Rico H, Revilla M, Villa LF, Hernandez ER, Alvarez de Buergo M, Villa M: Body composition in children and Tanner's stages: A study with dual-energy x-ray absorptiometry. Metabolism 1993; 42:967–970.

Dr. Gudrun Veldre, MSc, Vanemuise 46, Institute of Zoology and Hydrobiology,
University of Tartu, 51014 Tartu (Estonia)
Tel. +372 7 375 835, Fax +372 7 375 830, E-Mail gveldre@math.ut.ee

Jürimäe T, Hills AP (eds): Body Composition Assessment in Children and Adolescents.
Med Sport Sci. Basel, Karger, 2001, vol 44, pp 85–103

A Century of Growth in Australian Children

Tim Olds, Jim Dollman, Kevin Norton, Nathan Harten

School of Physical Education, Exercise and Sport Studies, University of
South Australia, Underdale, SA, Australia

It has been a consistent finding of studies from many parts of the world
that the height and mass of children have been increasing over the last 100–150
years [1]. A review of 113 reports of increases in height in 14 countries since
1860 shows an average increase of 1.35 ± 1.19 cm·decade^{-1}. The average increase in mass from 114 reports from 9 countries was 1.07 ± 0.92 kg·decade^{-1}
[Harten and Olds, unpubl. data]. There has been some speculation that in
recent years the secular increase in height and mass has slowed or stopped in
some parts of the world [2, 3].

Although there have been many large anthropometric surveys of Australian schoolchildren from 1897 onwards, the earliest complete raw dataset
of Australian schoolchildren was the result of a survey conducted in 1985 [4].
The authors have been able to reconstruct partial individual data from surveys
in 1937, 1954 and 1970 from frequency tables. Where raw data have been
discarded, available summary statistics are often lacunary or inappropriate.
For example, no standard deviations are available before 1937, and means and
standard deviations are typically used to describe mass, which usually shows
a strong positive skew. Even when raw data are available, comparison is con-
founded by methodological differences in measurement techniques and the
use of different and inappropriate scaling procedures. As a result, extensive
primary data treatment is necessary before meaningful comparisons can be
made and trends examined.

There have been very few large-scale studies taking direct measurements
of fatness (for example, skinfolds or hydrodensitometry), and with skinfold
measurements the large technical error of measurement can swamp small
secular drifts. Consequently, great reliance is placed on measurements of mass

and mass-for-height indices which provide only indirect estimates of fatness. The observed increases in mass and mass-for-height measures must also be interpreted against a background increase in height, and therefore an expected increase in mass. A primary concern is how to decide whether the increase in mass has been disproportionate in relation to the increase in height.

The aim of this paper was to review studies of the height and mass of Australian children since 1901 in an attempt to address three questions:

(1) Has the secular trend in height and mass slowed or stopped in Australia?

(2) Has mass increased disproportionately to height?

(3) Has there been a change in the distribution of mass?

Methods

Has the Secular Trend Slowed or Stopped?

Sources. The data reported in this paper are derived from 41 reports (62 datasets) on 5- to 16-year-old (at last birthday) Australian children collected between 1901 and 1997. The total number of subjects was 517,203, consisting of 268,546 boys and 248,657 girls. Of these, individual data were available for 32,510 boys and 30,894 girls. Data from reports relating exclusively to individual ethnic groups (for example, Australian aboriginals) were excluded.

Primary Data Treatment. To compare studies, a primary data treatment system was put in place. This is illustrated in figures 1 and 2. Height was standardised to waking height. Where stretch was not applied, height was corrected for the diurnal decrease, using an equation derived from a recent study of Australian schoolchildren [5]:

$$S = \ln(-0.00216T + 2.7173),$$

where S is stature as a fraction of waking stature, and T is the number of hours after waking. Because heights are very nearly normally distributed, the mean values were taken as the medians.

Mass was standardised to mass in light clothing (for example, gym wear with no shoes). Corrections were first made for clothing based on measurements of present and historical clothing items. Mass is not normally distributed, hence studies which report only the means and SDs make it difficult to estimate the median values. A log-transformation procedure was used to derive the probable median. The relationship between the mean of raw values and the mean of the log-transformed values for age- and sex-specific data slices was derived from existing raw datasets from 1954, 1970, 1985 and 1997. There was a very tight curvilinear fit:

$$L = -0.00031M^2 + 0.05105M + 2.114$$

$$r = 0.994, \ n = 52, \ p \leq 0.0001, \ RMSR = 0.0121$$

Where L is the mean of the log-transformed scores, and M is the mean of the raw scores. This allowed an estimation of the mean of the log-transformed values (and hence, by anti-

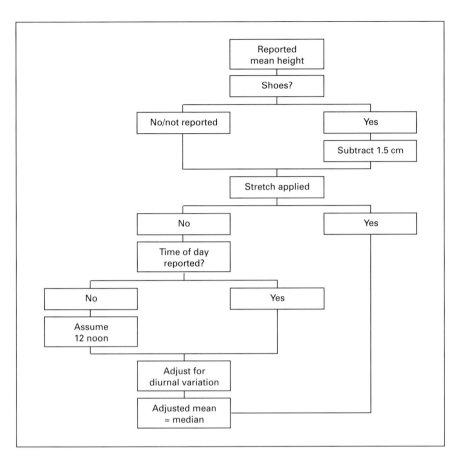

Fig. 1. Primary data treatment procedures for reported heights.

logging, the median) from the mean of the raw values. Estimated medians, as well as the reported and actual medians, were used in the examination of trends in changes in mass, but not in the analysis of trends in mean-median differences (see below).

Regressions of Changes in Mass and Height against Year of Study. Unweighted median values for height and mass for each year group from age 5 to age 16 (at last birthday) were regressed against year of measurement to determine linear trends. To see if the rate of change in height and mass has slowed, regressions were calculated over a rolling forty-year period (i.e. 1900–1940, 1910–1950), and the slopes compared.

Has Mass Increased Disproportionately to Height?

Three approaches have been used to judge whether the rate of increase in mass has been disproportionate to the rate of height increase: (1) the use of allometric exponents; (2) comparison at the same maturational age; (3) comparison at the same height.

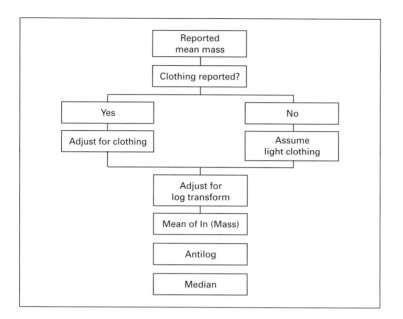

Fig. 2. Primary data treatment procedures for reported masses.

The Use of Allometric Exponents. Mass-for-height indices are most commonly exponential functions of the sort Mass=aHeight^b, where b is the allometric exponent. The most familiar of these indices is the Body Mass Index, where b=2. The Rohrer Index (b=3) is also used, reflecting a geometrical similarity system. These indices have often been used as a surrogate for fatness in children, using either arbitrary cut-offs or percentile values as limits for obesity.

The use of allometric mass exponents with children is problematic. Empirical examination of datasets shows that the exponent changes with age, peaking just before puberty at values of 3 or more, and then declining into adulthood before settling at values of 1.5–1.8. Figure 3 shows the mass exponents for girls aged 7–15 from a 1985 Australian survey and the NHANES III survey in the US [6]. While both follow a similar pattern, the American data yield consistently higher exponents. According to which exponent one chooses, mass-for-height can be judged to have increased, decreased or remained the same. Consider the data on the average 10-year-old girl presented in table 1. According to which exponent is chosen, we might conclude that mass for height has increased (BMI), stayed the same (mass$^{2.8}$, the empirically determined exponent) or fallen (Rohrer).

There is a second problem with using mass-for-height indices, associated with earlier maturation. The 12-year-old girl today is maturationally closer to the 15-year-old from the beginning of the century. Should the allometric exponent for 12-year-olds (2.8) or for 15-year-olds (1.9) be used?

It is therefore difficult to make judgment about increases in obesity based on mass-for-height indices. The best one can do is to make conservative judgments about appropriate exponents (that is, choose high exponents) when comparing datasets from different periods,

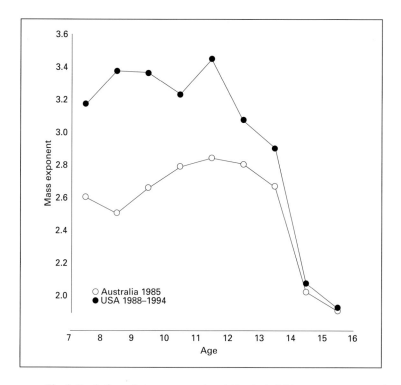

Fig. 3. Evolution of mass exponents relative to height across age groups based on data from the NHANES III survey, and the Australian Anthropometric DataBase.

Table 1. Mass, height and mass-for-height indices for the average 10-year-old girl in 1961 and 1985

Year	1961	1985
Mass, kg	31.6	34.0
Height, cm	136.7	140.3
BMI	16.9	17.3
Mass·height$^{-2.8}$	13.2	13.2
Rohrer Index	12.4	12.3

and look at the evolution of mass exponents over time. When exponents increase from one time period to another, the most likely explanation is that the shape of the population has changed – that is, they have become fatter. However, an increase in the mass exponent may also, depending upon which part of the age curve we are dealing with, reflect a maturational shift, or conceivably an increase in nonfat compartment masses.

Comparing Masses at Equivalent Heights. If the median mass at any given height is similar across studies, then mass is probably not increasing disproportionately. If mass at any given height is increasing over time, it is likely that children are becoming fatter. Unfortunately, there are very few datasets before 1985 which provide both mass and height for individual subjects. To assure reliability within each height band, the sample size must be fairly large and/or the height band quite wide. Because of height increases, not all height bands are comparable across all studies. Furthermore, this approach does not take into account maturational shifts. In this paper, we will compare median masses in given height bands for 13-year-olds between 1937, 1985 and the 1990s.

The Effects of Earlier Maturation. The age of menarche has been declining by about 4 months every decade over the course of this century, and the age at which boys' voices break may be decreasing by 2.5 months every decade [2]. In an effort to decide whether earlier maturation alone could account for increases in mass, estimated age at menarche was calculated using a regression equation based on a series of international studies reported in Norton and Olds [7]. The equation used was:

$$\text{Menarcheal age} = 81.1 - 0.0347 \text{ Year}$$

where Year is the chronological year. Age was then expressed as a percentage of estimated menarcheal age. The median masses at these adjusted ages reported from a series of studies of girls aged 7–12 were then compared to the median masses for age for girls aged 7–12 based on a large national Australian survey in 1985 [4]. If maturation can explain all the changes in mass in these girls, all the datapoints should fall close to the 1985 growth curve.

Has There Been a Change in the Distribution of Mass?

Increases in mass or mass-for-height can be due to a uniform shift affecting all members of the population, or the result of differential increases selectively affecting different members, either due to varying genotypically mediated susceptibilities or to differential exposure to permissive environments [8]. These different types of distributional shift result in characteristic patterns of change in summary statistics. If values at the higher percentiles are becoming progressively more extreme, the coefficients of variation and the differences between the mean and median values will increase over time. These summary statistics can therefore be regarded in the absence of raw data as markers of this type of distributional shift.

Coefficients of variation for mass, and the mean-median differences, were taken directly from the literature or calculated from raw data. Mean-median differences (MMDs) were expressed as a fraction of the means. Because there was a strong inverted-U relationship between CV and age, and the MMD and age (both peaking at peripubertal years), and because the age of the sample groups was positively correlated with the year of the study, quadratic regressions were fitted to the CV-age and MMD-age datapoints, the residuals calculated and plotted against year. A positive slope would signal increasing skew over time.

Results

Has the Secular Trend Slowed or Stopped?

There was a strong linear relationship between the year of the study and height and between year and mass across all age groups and both sexes, with a median correlation coefficient of 0.87. For height, the increases ranged from

Table 2. Increases in height and mass in Australian children between 1901 and 1997

Age	Boys		Girls	
	height cm·decade^{-1}	mass kg·decade^{-1}	height cm·decade^{-1}	mass kg·decade^{-1}
5	0.46	0.29	0.58	0.34
6	0.44	0.27	0.59	0.36
7	0.73	0.41	0.78	0.47
8	0.82	0.56	0.91	0.63
9	0.91	0.73	0.93	0.76
10	0.99	0.76	1.13	0.96
11	1.00	0.96	1.03	1.06
12	0.97	1.03	1.17	1.28
13	1.46	1.40	1.01	1.21
14	1.52	1.59	1.15	1.47
15	1.66	1.97	0.65	1.06
16	1.10	1.63	0.57	1.01

0.44 cm·decade^{-1} for 6-year-old boys to 1.66 cm·decade^{-1} for 15-year-old boys. For mass, the range was from 0.27 kg·decade^{-1} for 6-year-old boys to 1.97 kg·decade^{-1} for 15-year-old boys (table 2). Increases were greatest in the peripubertal years.

The rolling 40-year averages for increases in height in 5- to 16-year-old boys are shown in figure 4. Height increases in girls and mass increases in both sexes showed similar patterns. There was a marked decline in the rate of increase between the periods 1940–1980 and 1950–1990 in both height and mass for both boys and girls, with occasional negative trends. Since then the increases have resumed.

Has Mass Increased Disproportionately to Height?

Comparing Masses Using Allometric Relationships. Given the arbitrary choice of appropriate allometric exponents, a conservative approach is to use higher values. Even when high-exponent indices (for example, the Rohrer Index, mass/height^3) are used, there has been an increase in mass for height. Table 3 shows changes in the mean BMI and Rohrer Index for 13-year-olds between 1937 and the 1990s in Australia. There has been a 4–8% increase in the mean Rohrer Index and a 10–15% increase in mean BMI over that period.

This increase is much more marked at the higher percentiles. In 1985 10% of 13-year-old girls and 19% of boys were above the 95th percentile value for

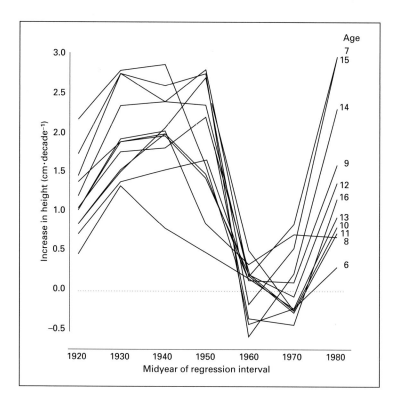

Fig. 4. Evolution of changes in height in Australian boys. Regressions of height against year were performed for each age group in moving 40-year intervals, starting with the period 1900–1940 and ending with 1960–2000. The slopes of the regressions are shown on the Y-axis in cm·decade^{-1}, plotted against the midpoint of each interval.

Table 3. Mean (SD) BMI and Rohrer Index values for 13-year-old Australian boys and girls in 1937, 1985 and the 1990s

Year	Boys		Girls	
	BMI	Rohrer Index	BMI	Rohrer Index
1937	17.30 (1.81)[a, b]	11.58 (1.23)[a, b]	18.15 (2.46)[b, c]	11.92 (1.66)[b, c]
1985	18.78 (2.86)[a, c]	12.17 (1.99)[a, c]	19.26 (2.69)[a]	12.42 (1.67)[a]
1990–1999	19.91 (3.46)[b, c]	12.55 (2.13)[b, c]	19.61 (2.69)[a]	12.39 (1.83)[a]

[a, b, c] Significantly different from 1937, 1985 and 1990–1999, respectively.

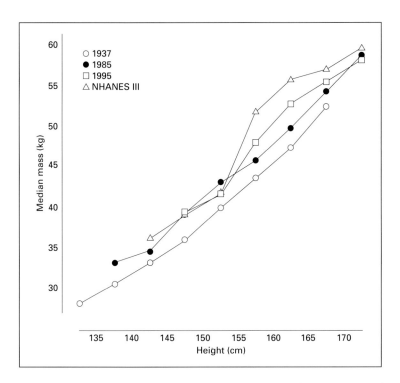

Fig. 5. Median masses of 13-year-old Australian boys in 1937, 1985 and 1990–1999 at different height bands. NHANES III data are shown for comparison.

BMI from the 1937 survey, and 9% and 13%, respectively, were above the 95th percentiles for the Rohrer Index. The corresponding figures for 1990–1999 were 11% (girls) and 34% (boys) for BMI, and 7% (girls) and 21% (boys) for the Rohrer Index. Therefore, even using very conservative measures of obesity, obesity has increased 2- to 4-fold in this age group.

There is also some evidence that mass exponents are increasing over time. In the 1937 sample, mass was proportional to height raised to the power 2.51 for 13-year-old boys and 2.44 for 13-year-old girls. By 1985, these had risen to 2.59 and 2.83, respectively. The corresponding figures in the NHANES sample are 3.36 and 2.90.

Comparing Masses at Given Heights. Figure 5 shows the median masses for a range of height bands for 13-year-old boys in 1937, 1985 and 1990–1999 in Australia. American data from the NHANES III survey in the US are shown for comparison. There is a general increase in mass at every height band as we move from 1937 to 1985 and 1990–1999, a trend which is exacerbated in the NHANES III sample. In the Australian samples, there has been over a

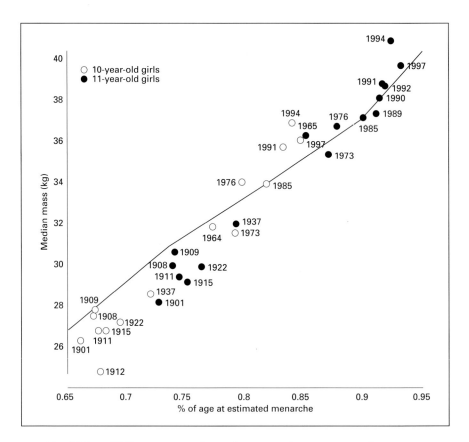

Fig. 6. The solid line represents the median masses for age, expressed as a percentage of estimated age at menarche (see text), from the 1985 Australian survey. The individual points represent the median masses of 10- and 11-year-old Australian girls (empty and filled circles, respectively) from studies between 1901 and 1997, plotted against age expressed as a percentage of estimated age at menarche.

60-year period an average increase in mass of about 3.5 kg, or about 8% of the median mass, at any height band. The pattern is similar for 13-year-old girls, with a 6% increase from 1937 to 1985, and a 10% increase between 1937 and the 1990s. The NHANES III 13-year-olds are on average 17% heavier at the same heights. This may represent increasing fatness, or earlier maturation associated with changing body shape. Because of the scarcity of matched height-weight datasets, comparisons in other age groups could not be made.

Comparing Masses at the Same Maturational Age. Figure 6 shows the median mass of 10- and 11-year-old Australian girls from studies between

1901 and 1997, plotted against chronological age expressed as a percentage of estimated age of menarche. The continuous line represents the median mass for age for girls aged 7–12 from the 1985 survey, where age is expressed as a percentage of estimated menarcheal age for 1985. The datapoints from the 32 studies fall quite close to the mass-for-age line from 1985, suggesting that the shift in median values can partly be explained by earlier maturation. However, a trend is also evident for values from earlier studies to fall below the line, and later studies to fall on or above the line. This suggests that even when allowance is made for maturation effects, girls from earlier studies are underweight relative to recent growth curves.

The same is not true for all age groups. The median mass of 13-year-old boys in 1937 is exactly the same (38 kg) as that of their 1985 maturational equivalents (assuming a maturation progression of 2.5 months per decade). The median mass of 13-year-old girls in 1937 (41.2 kg) is considerably greater than their 1985 maturational equivalents (37 kg at 11.45 years).

Has There Been a Change in the Distribution of Mass?

Figure 7 shows changes in the distribution of mass in Australian 13-year-olds from 1937 to 1995, along with the current US distribution. The graphs show an increasing positive skew.

This is confirmed by an analysis of values at specific percentiles (fig. 8). When masses are expressed as a percentage of the masses at the corresponding percentiles in 1954, there is very little change between 1954 and 1970. Mass has increased between 1970 and 1985 by about 3%, but the increase is fairly even across all percentile bands. When we compare the 1985 data to 1990–1995, however, the increase at the higher percentiles is much greater than that at the lower percentiles. There is only a 3% increase at the 10th percentile, but a 15% increase at the 90th percentile.

There is a strong linear relationship between age-corrected CV for mass and year in boys ($r = 0.75$, $p \leq 0.0001$, $n = 195$) and girls ($r = 0.48$, $p \leq 0.0001$, $n = 179$), showing that the CV for mass has increased over time. The relationship between raw CVs and year is significant for every age group (median $r = 0.66$). The evolution of MMDs is less strong, reaching significance in boys ($r = 0.37$, $p \leq 0.0001$, $n = 120$), but not in girls ($r = 0.05$, ns).

Discussion

In this paper we have attempted to piece together the shards of data available in an effort to recreate a century of growth in Australian children. Overall, the height and mass of children have been increasing in an approxi-

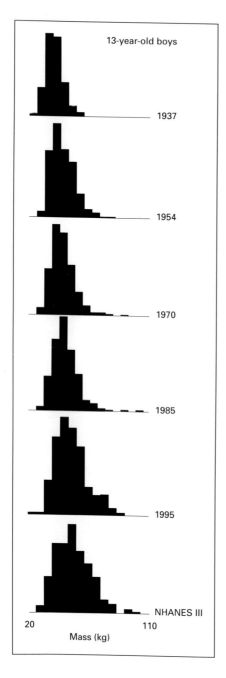

Fig. 7. Distribution of masses in Australian 13-year-olds from 1937 to 1995, along with the current US distribution.

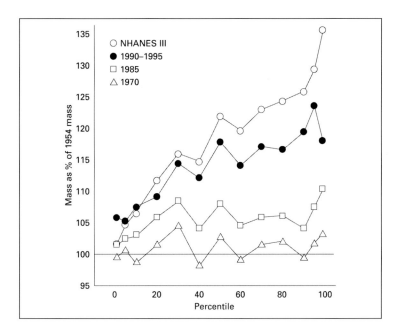

Fig. 8. Masses for 13-year-old boys in 1970, 1985, and 1990–1999, expressed as a percentage of the masses at the corresponding percentiles in 1954.

mately linear fashion by about 1.3 cm·decade^{-1} and 1.2 kg·decade^{-1}, similar to the overall trends reported in other studies [for example, 1].

Has the Secular Trend Slowed or Stopped?

Based on 40-year rolling regressions, the rate of increase of height and mass appeared to slow in Australia between the mid-1950s and the mid-1980s. Since then, however, the rate of increase appears to have accelerated again. Between 1900 and 1985, for example, the average rate of increase in height for 10- to 11-year-olds was 1.02 cm·decade^{-1}. compared to 2.56 cm·decade^{-1} in the period 1985–1997. The corresponding figures for 8- to 9-year-olds are 0.93 and 2.03 cm·decade^{-1}. There is therefore no evidence that the secular trend is currently slowing in Australia. The slowing of the rate of increase of height and mass from the mid-1950s to mid-1980s may be associated with two large waves of immigration from southern Europe and later from South-East Asia. In both cases, immigrant children were much shorter than Australian-born children.

Has Mass Increased Disproportionately to Height?

There have been a number of reports of a secular trend in fatness in children from around the world. US children showed a significant increase in

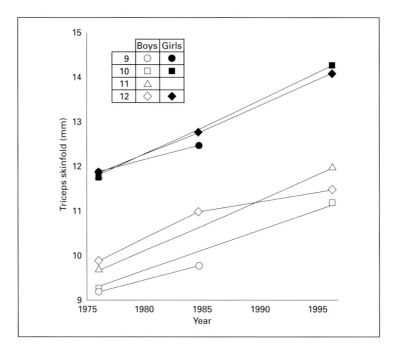

Fig. 9. Evolution of the triceps skinfold thickness in 9- to 12-year-old Australian boys and girls between 1976 and 1997.

triceps and subscapular skinfold thicknesses between 1963 and 1987 [9]. A recent report on Canadian youth [10] compared skinfold data on 10- to 16-year-old boys and 8- to 13-year-old boys between surveys in 1964–1973 and 1991–1997. Tanner and Whitehouse [11] found an increase in the triceps skinfolds of British boys between 1962 and 1973. In Australia, there has been at least one report of a disproportionate increase in mass in relation to height in school-aged males since 1986 [12]. More recent reports from the US show continued increases in skinfold thicknesses in 5- to 17-year-old children [13].

An examination of limited Australian skinfold data reveals a similar pattern. Figure 9 shows the evolution of triceps skinfold thicknesses in 9- to 12-year-old Australians between 1976 and 1997. There has been a consistent increase of about 1 mm·decade^{-1} in each age and gender slice.

Has Mass Increased Beyond Allometric Expectancy? The use of the BMI as a marker of increases in fatness is children is questionable given the actual allometric relationship between mass and height at these ages. In fact, it is difficult to mount a convincing case for any particular exponent. Using conservative metrics such as the Rohrer Index, there has still been a dispropor-

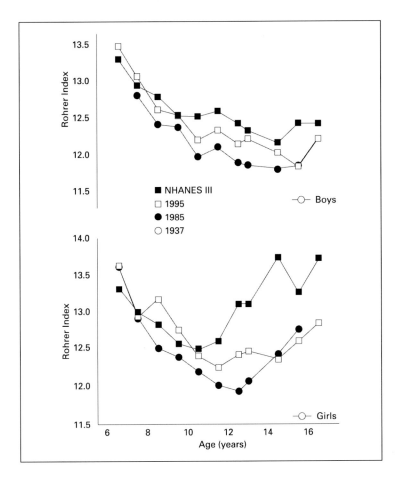

Fig. 10. Changes in the Rohrer Index between 1937 and 1997 in Australia, and US data from the NHANES III sample.

tionate increase in mass relative to height. Figure 10 shows the evolution of the Rohrer Index between 1937 and the 1990s in Australia, and in the US. There has been a consistent rise across most age bands. This is consistent with findings from the Bogalusa Heart Study [13] which documents increases in both BMIs and the Rohrer Index between 1973 and 1994, accelerating in the latter half of that period.

Has Mass Increased for Any Given Height? Comparison of data over the 60 years from 1937 shows a clear increase in mass in any given height band for 13-year-olds. Similar though less consistent patterns are found in comparisons over shorter time spans. In 10-year-old girls between 1985 and 1995, for example, mass at any given height has increased by 0–15%, with larger differences among taller girls.

Can Earlier Maturation Explain the Increase in Mass? Trying to assess masses at equivalent maturational ages is bedevilled with gross approximations of the rate of maturational progression, small sample numbers, inconsistent results according to the age group chosen, and possible confounding effects of social factors such as slimming behaviours. However, increases in mass in age groups beyond puberty suggest that not all increases can be explained by earlier maturation.

Has There Been a Change in the Distribution of Mass?

There have been few population data on changes in the distribution of fatness. When the distributions of triceps skinfold values in British boys taken by Tanner and Whitehouse in 1962 and 1973 are compared [11], there is little difference at the 5th and 50th percentiles, but a large increase at the 97th percentile. A recent American analysis of the NHANES surveys has also found evidence of increasing positive skews in measures of mass and mass-for-height [14], a finding reproduced in the Bogalusa study [13]. Paediatric obesity clinics both in Australia and overseas have often reported that they are seeing more children and that their level of obesity is becoming greater [15, 16]. Comparisons of skinfold and mass for height data on American children between 1965 and 1976–1980 [17] and between 1973 and 1994 [13] show increases in the incidence of obesity and superobesity. Finally, recent Danish data [18] show stable BMIs at the lower percentiles since 1930, but clear increases at the upper part of the distribution.

However, small shifts in the mean of a distribution can have very large effects at the extremes. A 1% increase in the mean (about a 400 g increase in mass in 10- or 11-year-olds) spread evenly across all members of the population will increase the number of children at or above the previous 99th percentile by 70%. A 2.5% increase will more than treble the number, and a 5% increase will increase it ninefold. Therefore, if criteria for obesity based on percentile cutoffs from earlier datasets continue to be used, the number of children with criterion-referenced obesity will increase dramatically, even if increases in mass have been moderate and uniform.

What Is Causing the Drift in Mass and Mass-for-Height?

There appears to have been a real increase in mass and mass-for-height in Australian children, particularly since 1985 [19], which selectively affects a subset of individuals. It is almost certain that this is due to an increase in fatness, and that similar trends are occurring in several developed countries. What factors might be behind these trends? The postwar period has been a period of major social change in Australia. It has seen the introduction of a wider range of sedentary leisure pursuits (for example, television and computer games). Data from the Australian Bureau of Statistics [20] reveal that between the 1960s and 1990s, car and television ownership per head of population doubled. In 1978, there were only two feature films available on video, and less than 3% of households had VCRs. By 1994, over 80% of households had a VCR and there were 33,000 films available. In addition, 18% of all households had a PC dedicated to games. Some, but not all, researchers have found significant associations between television viewing and obesity in children [21].

At the same time, changing family structures have made it harder for parents to share active leisure with their children. Between 1983 and 1992, there was a 50% increase in the number of one-parent families where the parent was in full-time employment. Of all couples with dependent children, 40.3% were both in full employment in 1983. By 1997, this had risen to 56.3%. In 1986, 49% of women with dependent children were in the workforce. The corresponding figure in 1996 was 59%. Not surprisingly, these shifts were accompanied by increases in the use of childcare: the percentage of children aged 0–5 in childcare doubled between 1984 and 1993. The dietary behaviour of Australians has also changed, with a 65% increase in household expenditure on eating out and takeaway food between 1984 and 1995. Changes in family structure were accompanied by economic shifts. The rich (essentially double-income households) became richer while the poor (single parents or unemployed) became poorer (the ratio of the 10th percentile income to 90% income fell by over 10% in the 10 years after 1983). There was therefore a large pool of people with insufficient resources, or time, or both, to actively engage with their children in recreational activities.

Concerns about safety and an unwillingness to leave children unsupervised, the cost of access to physical recreation facilities, and the breakdown of the extended family due to job insecurity and increased mobility all mean that there is less opportunity for children to play actively. There is increasing competition for time in the school curriculum, so there is less time and less expertise in schools for implementing structured physical activity programs. In the US, daily enrolment in physical education classes fell from 42% in 1991 to 25% in 1995.

Some researchers [8, 18] believe that a subset of the population is predisposed to obesity given appropriate environmental conditions. They suggest that the so-called 'thrifty gene' complex has evolved as an evolutionary strategy for dealing with irregular food supply – storing food rapidly during times of plentiful supply to counter times of shortage. However, most Australians now live in a milieu of abundance. This, coupled with a social environment which discourages physical activity, may allow the gene complex to express itself.

While speculative, such selective impacts would be consistent with the observed pattern of increase in mass: a major gene susceptible to environmental influences modifying its expression may characterise the higher mass percentiles.

Acknowledgments

The authors would like to acknowledge the assistance of Darren Burgess for making recent raw data and early studies available. This research has been partly supported by the Australian Financial Markets Children's Fund.

References

1   Meredith HV: Findings from Asia, Australia, Europe and North America on secular change in mean height of children, youths and young adults. Am J Phys Anthropol 1976;44:315–326.

2   Roche AF: Secular trends in stature, mass and maturation; in Roche AF (ed): Secular Trends in Human Growth, Maturation, and Development. Chicago, Society for Research in Child Development, 1979, pp 3–27.

3   Pheasant S: Bodyspace. London, Taylor & Francis, 1996.

4   Pyke J: Australian Health and Fitness Survey. Adelaide, ACHPER, 1987.

5   Burgess D, Olds TS, Norton KI: Evolution of the height and mass of Australian children. Proc Australian Conf Science and Medicine in Sport, Canberra, ASMF, 1996, pp 94–95.

6   US Department of Health and Human Services, National Centre for Health Statistics: NHANES III Reference Manuals and Reports (CD-ROM). Hyattsville, Centers of Disease Control & Prevention, 1996.

7   Norton KI, Whittingham N, Carter JEL, Kerr D, Gore C, Marfell-Jones MJ: Measurement techniques in anthropometry; in Norton KI, Olds TS (eds): Anthropometrica. Sydney, UNSW Press, 1996, pp 25–75.

8   Price RA, Ness R, Sørensen TIA: Changes in commingled Body Mass Index distributions associated with secular trends in overweight among Danish young men. Am J Epidemiol 1991;133:501–510.

9   Ross JG, Pate RR, Lohman TG, Christenson GM: Changes in the body composition of children. JOPERD 1987;58:74–77.

10   Thompson AM, Mirwald RL, Bailey DA: Secular trend and gender differences in adiposity in childhood and adolescence (abstract). Med Sci Sports Exerc 1999;31(suppl):S319.

11   Tanner JM, Whitehouse RH: Revised standards for triceps and subscapular skinfolds in British children. Arch Dis Child 1975;50:142–145.

12   Wilcken DEL, Lynch JF, Marshall MD, Scott RL, Wang XL: Relevance of body mass to apolipoprotein levels in Australian children. Med J Aust 1996;164:22–25.

13   Freedman DS, Srinivasan SR, Valdez RA, Williamson DF, Berenson GS: Secular increases in relative weight and adiposity among children over two decades: The Bogalusa Heart Study. Pediatrics 1997;99:420–426.

14   Troiano RP, Flegal KM: Overweight children and adolescents: Description, epidemiology, and demographics. Pediatrics 1998;101:497–504.

15   Hirata K: Changes in the body type of Japanese pupils from 1955–1975; in Shephard RJ, Lavallée H (eds): Physical Fitness Assessment. Springfield, Thomas, 1978, pp 263–272.

16   Naughton G, Gibbons K: Key into life. Proc 21st Biennial National/International ACHPER Conf. Adelaide, ACHPER, 1998, pp 98–100.

17   Gortmaker SL, Dietz WH, Sobol AM, Wehler CA: Increasing pediatric obesity in the United States. AJDC 1987;141:535–540.

18 Sørensen TIA: Genetic and environmental factors related to the development of obesity in young-sters; in Froberg K, Lammert O, St Hansen H, Blimkie C (eds): Children and Exercise XVIII. Odense, Odense University Press, 1997, pp 37–48.

19 Dollman J, Olds TS, Norton KI, Stuart DB: The evolution of fitness and fatness in 10–11-year-old Australian schoolchildren. Ped Exerc Sci 1999;11:108–121.

20 Castle I (ed): Australian Social Trends. Canberra, Australian Bureau of Statistics, 1997, pp 164–167.

21 Gortmaker SL, Dietz WH, Cheng LWY: Inactivity, diet and the fattening of America. J Am Diet Assoc 1990;90:1247–1256.

Tim Olds, PhD, School of Physical Education, Exercise and Sport Studies,
University of South Australia, Holbrooks Rd, Underdale, SA 5032 (Australia)
Tel. +61 8 8302 6709, Fax +61 8 8302 6658, E-Mail tim.olds@unisa.edu.au

Jürimäe T, Hills AP (eds): Body Composition Assessment in Children and Adolescents.
Med Sport Sci. Basel, Karger, 2001, vol 44, pp 104–114

....

Body Image and Its Relationship with Body Composition and Somatotype in Adolescents

Franco Viviani

Higher Institute of Physical Education of Bologna, Padua Section and Faculty of
Psychology, University of Padua, Italy

There is more reason in your body than in your better knowledge
Nietzsche: 'Also spracht Zaratustra'

When studying the body we still utilise the Cartesian model [1]: as we cannot advance scientifically if we do not use the order of quantity, that is, that of the number, we must reduce the body to the dimension of an organism, a sum of organs. The body as a 'thing' then, can be investigated, tested, cured. The different and sometimes very sophisticated body composition (BC) techniques currently being employed are thus an extension of the mechanistic interpretation of the world. As long as the study of the body is confined to the thorough investigation of its constituent parts, no particular problems arise, but as soon as other body aspects are touched (such as those in relation to the Self), the problematic and mysterious relationships existing between body and mind come to the forefront. The potential for this to occur is heightened when the mechanistic vision shuns a substantial element: human creativity. The object of our scrutiny is, in fact, a complete, thinking human being in the environment. It is not an anatomo-physiological system isolated in a controlled laboratory setting. This objective has the wise and reasonable pretence of not being an object, but a *subject*. Clearly, the study of the human body is undertaken differently by an anatomist and a psychologist but that the approaches used are distantly related. Sometimes it is difficult to imagine how such scientists could carry on a reasonable dialogue even at the level of decision-making and agreement on the language to be used. The present paper attempts to clarify whether a more realistic approach among different scientific mentalities, methodologies and languages is advisable. This is bearing in mind that many philosophers argue that 'a complete prediction (in human body studies) is, in principle, not possible, no matter how sophisticated the methods of empirical science become' [2, p. 279].

Body Composition, Somatotype and BI

Two main models are used in the study of BC. The biochemical model uses in vitro and in vivo methods in adolescence, but is limited by the small number of subject studied. The other model is more related to application (and thus used by fitness centers, clinics or nutrition settings), which mainly adopt the two-compartment model (lean/fat). The latter approach is more holistic but does not furnish information on the differences occurring with growth and maturation in adolescents [3].

In relation to somatotype, if an anthropometrist wishes to interact meaningfully with a psychologist, it would be advantageous for him to affirm that somatotype is a *Gestalt*. Conceptually, and in a similar way to how early configurationists defiantly confronted the perceptual phenomena, the body is not seen as a juxtaposition or addition of its constituent parts, but rather globally, as it organizes itself in structures according to the biological instructions. This approach to the study of a body is also holistic. Somatotype permits an overall and concise view of a body only but cannot answer all questions related to physique. Somatotype is not causal, but changes occurring in a physique 'reflect the effects rather than the cause' [4, p. 349].

If a psychologist wants to explain to an anthropometrist some aspects of Self, such as body image (BI), he should first affirm that in the latter three main components converge: the *perceptual* (related to sensory and visuo-spatial judgements), *cognitive* (referred to thought processes and culturally mediated thinking styles) and *affective* (an aspect more directly connected to emotions and attitudes). Therefore BI is a multidimensional construct and much more holistic than the two aforementioned ones [5]. Here the body is no longer physique, nor a lean-fat hardware, but it becomes a light and shade representation whose boundaries are socially mediated.

It could be particularly useful for those studying BC and researchers to better understand the main psychosocial issues of relevance in adolescence. Benefits may include a comprehension of differences between adolescents and adults and the relationship between mental constructs and some anthropometric measurements. Psychometric tests (with the central focus of describing and quantifying the internal representations of Self and others) could give more useful insights to better assess human physique. The challenge would be to design more adequate, sophisticated and integrated tools for the study of the human body.

The Body and the Self

The construction of the Self and its representations are important topics for cognitive psychologists as different influences are believed to be at work for the various ages of the life cycle. Early in life the Self depends upon self-image, an ecologically linked percept, whose development is psycho-physio-logically related to our visual interaction with the environment [6]. Later on, the Self becomes more and more aware of the 'significant others' found in the environment and becomes a 'social being', able to build continuously re-arranged feedbacks and feed-forwards with the others. This is essential for survival, as human evolution has progressed by means of both cooperation and competition [7]. It is believed that self-recognition begins from approximately 18 to 24 months of age and self-awareness follows [8]. In the ontogenesis of self-conception, a basis is offered by a sense of personal agency, which has been evolutionarily connected to life in an arboreal habitat, where a constant vigilance of the body mass with respect to the arboreal support was required. Increasing evidence from studies carried out in primates shows that humans extend and elaborate their precocial onset of self-awareness [9]. This is a strategy that permits them to cope with a complex interpersonal milieu. Bodily/gestural imitation and self-recognition belongs to kinesthetic-visual matching, that is 'the capacity for matching between the kinesthetic, proprioceptive, and somasthetic sensations of body widths and heights'. This does not help individuals to be more precise in estimating BI, probably because of the imprecise awareness of their body dimensions and their desire to grow [10]. Experience, gender, person-ality, environment and so on are therefore implied in the building of BI and they are inextricably connected to form a dynamic unison.

Reflexive indicators (such as self-evaluation or self-examination) have been suggested [6]; together with evaluation indicators (signs of being satisfied or dissatisfied with the body), social-referent indicators (those legitimising or homologating the individual) and positional indicators, which permit the indi-vidual to locate him/herself in space or the social context. In research, two main aspects of BI are distinguished: the accuracy with which body size is estimated and the feelings shown in relation to the body (satisfaction/ dissatisfaction): for this reason not all the indicators are used, this is particu-larly the case in studies of adolescents.

Due to the wide range of procedures available for the assessment of BI, results are often misleading and potentially confusing. A number of extensive reviews of the methodologies used in the assessment of BI have been published [11–14].

Body Image in Adolescents

From birth, a child takes 10 years to develop its own body awareness. The construction of a mental image follows and, subsequently, a certain sense of equilibrium is reached between sense of identity and that of continuity. In adolescence this order is subverted, the child is obliged to work, to find new equilibria and is sometimes disturbed by the fact that a gap exists between the speeds at which somatic and psychological transformations occur [15]. Rapid physical changes result in the adolescent questioning the system which, up to the time of change, had regulated the individual relationships with his/her own body, those with other individuals or groups, those with activities or objects and with social institutions. Previous arrangements appear, at a certain point of his/her personal evolution, to be no longer valid [16]. Gender differences also occur and those not directly linked to growth and development (like the psychological ones) are probably connected to the fact that boys, in contrast to girls, realise that their body fully belongs to them. Often, girls appraise that because of probable future motherhood, their bodies are not completely their own, but somehow a 'social body'. This could explain some behavioural gender differences and others linked to the body. For example, boys are more concerned with stature, muscular and sexual development (low height and weight are most worrying to them), while girls consider excessive height and weight values as being most unbecoming [17].

It is believed that self-concept (very seldom used as a synonym for self-esteem) evolves during adolescence (at least in the Western culture) from an infantile manner (as it is projected towards the exterior and is considered in physical terms by its recipient) to an adult one (the so-called 'real self'). This is internalised and is more mental than physical. The adolescent Self is, in this manner, named 'ideal self' [18]. It is clear that disturbances of such cognitive construct occur at this age and mainly affects two aspects: the perceptual distortion in the estimation of body dimensions (the person is not able to correctly evaluate his/her body dimension) and the subjective evaluation of attitudes and cognition (the state of dissatisfaction with the body: this has a more affective meaning). This dychotomy has permitted two main research areas to be developed. The first, using instruments such as mirrors and sets of figurines, asks the subject to estimate his/her own body or body part boundaries. The second, more centred in the affective dimension, asks the subject his/her feelings of satisfaction/dissatisfaction with his/her own body.

Adult women value their appearance more than males [19], particularly experiencing more weight-related concerns expecially when young and middle-aged [5]. With advancing age, despite the tendency for weight gain, independence and self-confidence increase [20], neuroticism decreases [21] and therefore the importance of appearance declines [22]. But what happens in adolescents?

Studies of Adolescents

The Brodie and Slade [23] study on pre- and post-pubescent English youngsters found that girls, independent of their pre- or post-pubescent status, show a clear desire to be thinner, even if the tendency to perceive themselves fatter than they were was slight. Pre-adolescents were more satisfied with their body aspect than post-adolescents. A number of comparative studies have been undertaken on anorexic patients and caution is needed in the interpretation of results [24]. In general terms, puberty is apparently unrelated to BI, even if pre-pubescent subjects are less dissatisfied, probably because they are less critical [23]. The trend to slenderness in girls portayed by the media is found in many developed societies. The aspiration for thinness affects Australian girls. Brisbane girls worried about weight and thinness [25] and they 'felt fat' 2.5 times more than their male counterparts. In 15-year-old Czech girls [26] BI was a motivating factor to participation in a more healthy life-style (even if large numbers attempted to lose weight using other passive means). This occurred to a lesser extent in Italian girls as well [27]. The trend was found in Italian art students (aged 14–19 years). In general, the girls' tendency towards dissatisfaction regarding their own body was quite high, whilst opposite results were found in males. Significant sex differences emerged for height, weight, complexion, buttocks, hips, legs, ankles, general physical appearance and muscular tone. The 'actual' and the 'perceived' body, calculated on the scores obtained by means of comparison with figurines test did not show significant differences for sex and age. Apparently, adolescents are conscious recipients of their own body [27].

The data relating to physical structure and self-evaluation is of some interest. Adolescent girls showed that self-esteem is related to body weight, as the higher the BMI, the lower the level of self-esteem [28]. Significant adults (such as coaches) appear to be an important source of influence for an aspect of Self more directly connected to performance, self-efficacy (SE). In Spanish boys and girls higher SE scores were found in those athletes who had a higher perception of the coach's competence [29]. A negative correlation was found between body fat and SE [30].

Boys who perceived themselves as mesomorphic referred to a greater personal value, feelings of confidence, self-acceptance with respect to peers self-perceived as being ecto- or endomorphs. In adults, endomorphy appears to stir up external negative perceptions (since characteristics such as laziness, slowness and carelessness are attributed to it), while ectomorph women are considered to be attractive [31]. Endomorphs are also believed to be responsible for their own condition [32]. High correlations between self-perception of ones own physical structure and a subscale of Physical Self-Efficacy Scale were found by Chang et al. [33]. Lean and tall subjects gave significant scores with respect to fat and short subjects. Males gave higher scores than females. Male adolescents (11–12 and 13–15 years old) showed significantly better scores in the SE test than females [34]. Both sexes showed that excessive weight negatively correlated with motor SE ($r = -0.27$, $p < 0.01$).

Pre-pubescent boys and girls practising sporting activities (individual or team sports) gave a higher score both for SE and on the self-concept scale than non-practising peers [35]. The increase in motor abilities and the acquisition of sport skills appear to contribute to the development of a better self-concept and lower anxiety in adults as well [36–38].

Body size estimation is seemingly unrelated to body fat measures [23], but the affective dimension looms as dissatisfaction with the body is clearer when the subject becomes aware of his/her body size and shape measures. In boys, body size estimation is unrelated to maturation [38]. When girls perceive themselves as being larger, they display a thinner ideal image [23], a discrepancy that the authors attributed to the trend shown in adult women. The larger the body is perceived, the more negative the BI that is formed. This is not surprising, as healthy, relatively slim adult women show the desire to be slimmer [13] or participate in slimming sessions [39].

The use of the Askevold test [40] has provided additional interesting results. This tool requires that a subject, standing in front of a wall (onto which a sheet of paper has previously been fixed), uses a pencil to mark the main anthropometric points of the torso that are touched, one by one, by the examiner who is standing behind the subject. With anthropometric instruments, the distances between the various points of the body are measured. In this way it is possible to obtain two values: one 'subjective' and one 'objective'. The comparison between the two permits a more realistic description and quantification of the discrepancies that exist between the subject's internal representations and the objective reality.

In general, adult subjects show a slightly smaller subjective area [41], but we found that adolescents tend to perceive themselves slightly larger than they are in reality. In a sample of high school students aged 12, 15 and 18 years of age, who where administered a version of the body cathexis [42], a physical self-efficacy scale and the Askevold test were administered, the two genders perceived their body in a different way. Differences were found at a cognitive and an emotional level, with discernible age differences. For body size estimate, 12-year-old boys and girls declared higher values for acromial, cristale and trochanter heights, at 15 years of age these measures were not different from the actual measures. At 18 years of age, males perceived wider measures than actual ones, while girls showed higher values for stature only. Boys exhibited a better SE than girls; the latter always expressed a higher dissatisfaction with their body when compared to males.

In another cross-sectional study carried out in junior and high school children aged 12–19 years [43], all subjects of both gender in all age groups displayed a wider subjective area than objective when submitted to the Askevold test. 12- to 13- and 14- to 15-year-old boys and girls showed a similar trend for BI, while at 16–17 and 18–19 years, differences between the genders emerged. Males perceived a body area close to the actual area while females showed greater discrepancies, a result that was interpreted as follows. Because of the emphasis of slenderness for women, their dissatisfaction with the body is enhanced. This sharpens their sensitivity towards their own body shape, thus determining an overestimation of the body area.

In general, apart from the competitive dimension, exercise seems to contribute towards a higher self-appraisal, a lower level of trait-anxiety and better SE and self-concept. This is well known for adult women as changes in one facet of self-concept provokes changes in other facet (occupational, physical and social) [44]. Results show that in 12- to 14-year-old students [36], and older adolescents (17–19), males always exhibit a better SE and a lower level of trait anxiety connected to motor situations than females [37]. Interestingly, non-professional adolescent female ballet dancers do not differ from average girls for bodily self-perception [45]. No differences occurred between adults and adolescents for SE and body cathexis (more linked to the affective dimension of BI). Endomorphy was weakly correlated to SE ($r = 0.27$) and body cathexis ($r = 0.24$). In monozygote (MZ) adult and adolescent twins the firstborn in a couple shows a higher affective perception of his/her own body, and a better performance in the dexterity test. This often happens because the firstborn in a MZ couple is the more extroverted twin. Sex differences emerged for the total and various regional areas of the Askevold test [46].

In another study, thirty 10- to 12-year-old highly trained boys practicing soccer football were compared to 30 'sedentary' boys, showed no particular anthropometric differences, but they strongly differed in the torso areas as soccer players perceived themselves as being significantly larger [47]. Another survey involving boy and girls practicing tennis (14-year-olds) and swimming (12–13-year-olds) [48], compared to sedentary peers did not display the same results, probably due to the wide range of differences in judging body dimensions found in the samples. A further study carried out on 20 amateurs and 20 highly trained basketball players aged 13.4 ± 1.0 years, compared to an age-matched control, all the boys showed a subjective area larger than the objective, but results were conflicting. The 'champions' revealed the highest discrepancy between the two areas, the amateurs the lowest [38]. No differences emerged for BI assessed by means of the figurines and other cognitive aspects, checked by means of the Raven progressive matrices.

Conclusions

The Self is a dynamic unit and BI is one of its most representative parts. As affirmed earlier, the body is part of the Self and should not be considered as hardware to be disassembled to understand it better. Rather, it is a unit in the environment and reacts with it. Studies on adolescents show that BI is not fixed. Working on it could become the cornerstone of changing attitudes and behaviors in relation to the physique for adolescents and adults. Due to the different approaches employed, a neglected field of study is that of the correlations existing between BI, BC and somatotype. This is ruinous in each of the applied fields in relation to eating disorders, where BI was claimed to be implacably fixed. With the improvements of techniques for the assessment of BC, students and researchers alike must realise that to fully understand the body, an appraisal of BI is essential. Further clinical interventions, for example on fat/lean subjects, or clinical applications such as bulimia or anorexia nervosa treatment must be addressed to both BC and BI to improve the effectiveness of the therapies. New studies should be carried out in order to modify BI, a premise for better achievements in clinical settings. Links between somatotype, BC, personality and behaviour are imagined, but the fact that it is not possible to demonstrate that unequivocal cause/effect relationships existing among them must not discourage such attempts. This is more valid for adolescents, who are often lacking in emotional education (the basis for an adequate construction of self-concept) which requires self-esteem (a positive consideration of him/herself) and self-acceptation (the self-admission of one's own negative aspects or weaknesses). According to the 'isochronic theory' of the French auxologist Olivier, an adolescent grows thoroughly, or from all points of view [49], therefore social and affective inputs are very important. An adolescent is prone to social dictates and absorbs the aesthetic and physical values found in the environment. He/she tends towards syncretism but, because of the number of the goals to be achieved in complex western societies (when 'social' adolescence finishes?), and the fading of passing rites (which makes long-term rewards – like healthy adult life – less important than short-term rewards), he/she sometimes fails, due to the weakness of his/her symbolic borders. As a consequence, the mass media dictates for slenderness in girls or muscularity in boys require acceptance. But stereotype acceptance, as warned by Sleet [50], influences personality and behaviour, as the expectancies required by the stereotype must be fulfilled.

It is possible to affirm that if relationships between psychological tests and the methodologies used to measure the physical body exist, they are more general than specific [51]. If anthropometrists and anatomists are required to take into consideration the cognitive, affective and perceptual dimensions of the body, another big effort is required of psychologists, to use reliable measures of psychological functioning. Only in this way will that gap existing between different researchers be filled.

References

1   Chomsky N: Aspects of the Theory of Syntax. Cambridge, MIT Press, 1965.
2   Kretchmar RS: Philosophic research in physical activity; in Thomas JR, Nelson JK (eds): Research Methods in Physical Activity. Champaign, Human Kinetics, 1996, pp 277–290.
3   Malina RM, Bouchard C: Growth, Maturation, and Physical Activity. Champaign, Human Kinetics, 1991.
4   Carter JEL, Heath BH: Somatotyping. Development and Applications. Cambridge, Cambridge University Press, 1990.
5   Rozin P, Fallon A: Body image, attitudes towards weight and misperception of the figure preferences of the opposite sex: A comparison of men and women of two generations. J Abnorm Psychol 1988; 97:342–345.
6   Neisser U: The roots of self-knowledge: Perceiving self, it, and thou; in Snodgrass JG, Thompson RL (eds): The Self Across Psychology. New York, Annals of the New York Academy of Sciences, 1997, vol 818, pp 19–33.
7   Gallup GG: Self-recognition: research strategies and experimental design; in Parker S, Mitchell R, Boccia M (eds): Self-Awareness in Animals and Humans. New York, Cambridge University Press, 1994, pp 35–50.
8   Povinelli DJ, Cant JGH: Arboreal clambering and the evolution of self-conception. Q Rev Biol 1995;70:393–421.
9   Mitchell RW: A comparison of the self-awareness and kinesthetic-visual matching theories of self-recognition: Autistic children and others; in Snodgrass JG, Thompson RL (eds): The Self Across Psychology. New York, Annals of the New York Academy of Sciences, 1997, vol 818, pp 39–62.
10 Viviani F, Bortoli L, Robazza C: Cognitive and emotional bodily self-perception in youngsters; in Vanfranchem-Raway R, Vanden Auweele Y (eds): Proceedings of the IXth European Congress on Sport Psychology. Brussels, European Federation of Sport Psychology, 1995, pp 1285–1290.
11 Cash TF, Brown TA: Body image in anorexia nervosa and bulimia nervosa: A review of the literature. Behav Modif 1987;11:87–521.
12 Brodie DA, Slade PD: The relationship between body image and body fat in adult women. Psychol Med 1988;18:623–631.
13 Brodie DA, Slade PD, Riley VJ: Sex differences in body image perception. Perc Motor Skills 1991; 72:73–74.
14 Thompson J: Body Image Disturbance: Assessment and Treatment. Psychology Practitioner Books. London, Pergamon Press, 1990.

15   Montecchi F, Magnani M: Anoressia o anoressie? Psichiatr Inf Adolesc 1996;3:677–688.

16   Stern D: The Interpersonal Word of the Infant. New York, Basic Books, 1985.

17   Speltini G: Inquietudini e paure nell'adolescenza. Bologna, Cappelli, 1982.

18   Harter S: The perceived competence scale for children. Child Dev 1982;53:87–97.

19   Pliner C, Chaiken S, Flett GL: Gender differences in concern with body weight and physical appearence over the lifespan. Pers Soc Psychol Bull 1990;16:263–277.

20   Helson R, Moane G: Personality change in women from college to midlife. J Pers Soc Psychol 1987;53:176–186.

21   Costa PT, McCrae RR: Personality in adulthood: A 6 year longitudinal study of self-report and spouse rating in NEO personality inventory. J Pers Soc Psychol 1988;54:853–863.

22   Thomas CD, Freeman RJ: The body esteem scale: Construct validity of female subscales. J Pers Assess 1990;54:204–221.

23   Brodie DA, Slade PD: Perception of body image; in Fu FH, Mee-Lee Ng (eds): Sports Psychology: Perspectives and Practices Towards the 21st Century. Kowloon, Hong Kong Baptist University, 1995, pp 35–62.

24   Button EJ, Fransella F, Slade PD: A reappraisal of body perception disturbance in anorexia nervosa. Psychol Med 1977;7:235–243.

25   Byrne NM, Hills AP: Assessment of eating practices in adolescents. Proc Nutr Soc Austr 1995;19:104.

26   Fialovà L: Body image as a motivation factor for healthy life; in Svoboda B, Rychtecky A (eds): Physical Activity for Life: East and West, South and North. Prague, Meyer & Meyer, 1995, pp 407–412.

27   Viviani F, Brentel G, Marchioro G, Vinante O, Gorghetto S: Some aspects of body image and self-perception in adolescents; in Byrne D (ed): Psychosomatics Medicine: Towards the Year 2000. Sydney, Abstract Book of the 14th World Congress on Psychosomatic Medicine, 1997.

28   Martin S: Self-esteem of adolescents girls as related to weight. Perc Mot Skills 1988;67:879.

29   Escartì A, Garcìa Ferriola A, Cervellò E: Relationships between the perception of the coaches competence with the physical self-efficacy and level motivation; in Serpa S, Alves J, Ferreira V, Paula-Brito A: Sport Psychology: An Integrated Approach. Proceedings of the VIIIth World Congress of Sport Psychology. Lisbon, Universidade Técnica de Lisboa, 1993, pp 215–217.

30   Balogun JA: The interrelationships between measures of physical fitness and self-concept. J Hum Mov Studies 1987;13:255–257.

31   Ryckman RM, Robbins MA, Gold JA: Male and female raters' stereotyping of male and female physiques. Pers Soc Psychol Bull 1989;15:244–249.

32   Jasper CR, Klassen ML: Stereotypical beliefs about appearance: Implications for retailing and consumer issues. Perc Mot Skills 1990;71:519–521.

33   Chang RCM, Fung L, Cheung SY: A study of physical self-efficacy and physique perception; in Giam CK, Chook KK, Teh KC (eds): Proceedings of the VIIth World Congress in Sport Psychology, Singapore, 1989, pp 46–47.

34   Viviani F, Bortoli L, Robazza C, Casagrande G: Somatotipo, concetto di sé e self-efficacy motoria in un gruppo di giovani. Movimento 1991;7:147–149.

35   Bortoli L, Robazza C, Viviani F, Voltan M: Sport influence on self-concept and self-efficacy in children; in Svoboda B, Rychtecky A (eds): Physical Activity for Life: East and West, South and North. Prague, Meyer & Meyer, 1995, pp 22–25.

36   Bortoli L, Robazza C, Viviani F, Saccardi S: Influences of sport experience on physical self-efficacy, anxiety and self-concept; in Serpa S, Alves J, Ferreira V, Paula-Brito A (eds): Sport Psychology: An Integrated Approach. Proceedings of the VIIIth World Congress of Sport Psychology. Lisbon, Universidade Técnica de Lisboa, 1993, pp 159–162.

37   Bortoli L, Robazza C, Viviani F, Pesavento M: Auto eficacia fisica, percepciòn corporal y ansiedad en hombres y mujeres. Actas del Congreso Cientifico Olimpico 1992. Màlaga, Instituto Andaluz del Deporte, 1996, vol 24, I, pp 239–242.

38   Viviani F, Lavazza A, Grassivaro Gallo P, Marchioro G, Gorghetto S, Vinante O: Body image changes in adolescents practicing and non-practicing physical activity; in Byrne D (ed): Psychosomatics Medicine: Towards the Year 2000. Abstract Book 14th World Congress on Psychosomatic Medicine, Sydney, 1997.

39 Casagrande G, Viviani F: A methodological approach to the assessment of the 'ideal body figure' in fat, obese and non-obese women; in Coetsee MF, Van Heerden HJ (eds): Proceedings of the International Council for Physical Activity and Fitness Research. Nutrition and Physical Activity. KwaDlangezwa, Department of Human Movement Science, University of Zululand, 1997, pp 70–75.

40 Askevold F: Measuring body image: Preliminary report of a new method. Psychother Psychosom 1975;26:71–77.

41 Robazza C: L'ipnosi nella preparazione mentale del'atleta: Sperimentazione con soggetti praticanti karate. Movimento 1990;6:76–81.

42 Secord PF, Jourard SM: The appraisal of body cathexis: Body cathexis and the self. J Consult Psychol 1953;17:343–347.

43 Viviani F, Bortoli L, Robazza C, Grassivaro Gallo P: Body image in adolescents subjects; in Coetsee MF, Van Heerden HJ (eds): Proceedings of the International Council for Physical Activity and Fitness Research. Nutrition and Physical Activity. KwaDlangezwa, Department of Human Movement Science, University of Zululand, 1997, pp 130–134.

44 Taylor ASJ, Paruk Z: Women and psychosocial implications of physical activity; in Coetsee MF, Van Heerden HJ (eds): Proceedings of the International Council for Physical Activity and Fitness Research. Nutrition and Physical Activity. KwaDlangezwa, Department of Human Movement Science, University of Zululand, 1997, pp 120–129.

45 Casagrande G, Viviani F, Bortoli L, Robazza C, Peloso M, Grassivaro Gallo P: Some morphological, physiological and psychological aspects in females practicing ballet dancing; in Viviani F, Casagrande G, Claessens AL (eds): Abstract book of the 1996 ICPAFR Symposium, 1996, pp 76.

46 Viviani F, Bortoli L, Robazza C, Pasqualinotto AP, Pasqualinotto AG, Casagrande G: Self-perception, morphological characteristics and physical abilities in monozygote twins; in Casagrande G, Viviani F (eds): Physical Activity and Health. Physiological, Behavioral and Epidemiological Aspects. Padua, Unipress, 1998, pp 91–96.

47 Viviani F: Body image in Italian junior male soccer players. AJPHERD 1996;2:143–148.

48 Viviani F, Grassivaro Gallo P: Body image in circumpubertal swimmers and tennis players. AJPHERD 1997;3:211–217.

49 Olivier G: Causes of biological differences among social classes. J Hum Evol 1979;8:813–816.

50 Sleet DA: Typecasting – Does your body type affects your personality? Shape 1982;2:40–42, 90–91.

51 Kane J: Personality, body concept and performance; in Kane J (ed): Psychological Aspects of Physical Education and Sport. London, Routledge & Kegan Paul, 1972, pp 91–127.

Franco Viviani, Department of General Psychology, University of Padua,
Via Venzia, 8, I–35131 Padova (Italy)
Tel. +39 049 8804668, Fax +39 049 8276600, E-Mail vyfra@hotmail.com

Jürimäe T, Hills AP (eds): Body Composition Assessment in Children and Adolescents.
Med Sport Sci. Basel, Karger, 2001, vol 44, pp 115–131

....

Gender and Activity Comparison of Body Composition among Australian Children

Timothy R. Ackland, Brian A. Blanksby

Department of Human Movement and Exercise Science, University of Western Australia,
Nedlands, WA, Australia

Data for this paper were derived from The University of Western Australia Growth and Development Study [1]. The aim of this project was to bring together a group of children who participated successfully in competitive swimming and tennis, and a group of similar age and socio-economic status who did not participate in regular sport. Previous studies had measured large numbers of subjects but they were not selected on the basis of athletic success. It was hoped that choosing youngsters who were successful in swimming and tennis might throw some light on any factor throughout growth that may indicate some reason for that success.

Swimming is a sport that involves training in a water medium; it takes place in a horizontal body position and uses both upper limbs and both lower limbs for propulsion through the water. In contrast, tennis is generally a unilateral sport, whereby one racquet arm plays a more dominant role than the non-racquet arm. Both lower limbs are required to move the body around the court and the activity takes place in an upright posture, more in line with everyday postures.

In this chapter we will present normative data for growth in morphology and adiposity of Australian adolescents (with respect to both chronological and biological age) and review some of the previously published research related to gender and activity group comparisons.

The Sample

This mixed longitudinal project commenced in November, 1981 with the selection of swimmers who were finalists in the Western Australian (W.A.) state swimming championships.

The subjects (n = 172) ranged in age from 8 to 12 years and trained intensively at an average frequency of five sessions per week. Competitive swimmers remained in this sample through-out the duration of the study provided they continued to compete in subsequent state championship events.

In May, 1982 a group of leading junior tennis players, aged 8–14 years (n = 172), were also selected. The younger participants were recommended by professional coaches, while the group of 11- to 14-year-old subjects was selected on W.A. state tournament results. The attainment of a regular quarter-final position was used as the criterion level of performance.

Male and female subjects aged 7–12 years were admitted into a non-competitive group (n = 257), based on the criterion that they were not involved in regular, formal training for a sport more than once per week. These subjects were monitored throughout the study in order to verify their adherence to this criterion. This group was chosen from schools which matched the socio-economic status of the swimmers and tennis players (schools rated as being located in high, medium or low socio-economic zones by the Australian Bureau of Statistics). Good retention of subjects for the complete investigation was a feature of this project (56% overall for the 5 years).

Procedures

Subjects were assessed at 6-monthly intervals, within a 2-week period, on a battery of tests that included pubescence, anthropometric, physical, physiological and psycho-social measurements.

Tester Competence and Reliability

With the exception of the pubescence assessment, which was performed by a medical practitioner, all testers were graduate and undergraduate students who were required to train in all of the testing protocols but become specialist testers for two areas. They were required to pass test-retest reliability trials in their two areas of special competence.

Pubescence Assessment

Subjects were examined by a medical practitioner of the same gender in a private room. Blood pressure and heart sounds also were checked and a maturity rating was made based on the five stages of adolescent development as described by Tanner [2]. The assessment for this study relied primarily on the amount and distribution of pubic hair, although genital development in males, and breast development in females, was used in cases of uncertainty [2].

Anthropometry and Body Composition

A series of 19 anthropometric variables were selected to monitor growth in dimensions of length, breadth and girth. The specific landmarks and measurement protocols used were based on the descriptions by Montague [3] and Hrdlicka [4], and since they vary slightly with the current ISAK standards [5], readers should be cautious when making direct comparisons with these data. All measures were made on the preferred side (whether right- or left-handed) of the body and landmarks were identified by two experienced anthropometrists for the full series of tests.

Adiposity was assessed by summing the triceps, subcapular, supra-iliac (similar to supra-spinale), abdominal and medial calf skinfolds. All skinfold measurements were taken on the preferred side of the body to the nearest 0.1 mm, using a Harpenden skinfold caliper. The procedure was repeated until two consecutive measures were made within 0.2 mm and the mean of these two values was then recorded. The relevant measurements from the anthropometric and skinfold tests also were used to calculate the somatotype according to the Heath-Carter method [6].

Normative Data

Though data have been published in the scientific literature with respect to age and gender norms for body dimensions and indices of adiposity, these data offer a unique insight to the growth process. This is because the normative data were derived from a mixed longitudinal survey and, while mean data are presented for each age, they are also stratified according to biological age via pubescence assessment. Similar data for other measurements in the test battery can be found in the literature [1]. Graphs of mean data in figures 1–3 comprised a minimum of 10 subjects in various stages of maturation as follows:

Males		Females	
Pre-adolescent	8–14 years	Pre-adolescent	8–12 years
PA stage 2	11–14 years	PA stage 2	10–13 years
PA stage 3	11–14 years	PA stage 3	11–13 years
PA stage 4	13–16 years	PA stage 4	12–16 years
PA stage 5	14–16 years	PA stage 5	13–16 years

Figure 1 displays mean values for stature with respect to gender and age categories for 8- to 16-year-old male and female subjects. As expected, the graphs for mean stature demonstrate an increased rate of growth for males at approximately 14 years of age and similarly, at approximately 12 years of age for females. It is clear from figure 1 that those subjects who mature early are taller than average. The later developers are smaller than average at each of the ages beyond 12 years for boys, and 10 years for girls. For example, at 14 years of age for the male sample, pre-adolescent subjects were 9.0 cm shorter than average, while subjects who had reached PA stage 5 were 12.5 cm taller than average. However, this disparity in stature between the various maturity groups for each age cohort of females was not so marked compared with the males.

Figure 2 displays mean values for body mass with respect to gender and age. Mean body mass demonstrates an increased rate of growth at approxi-

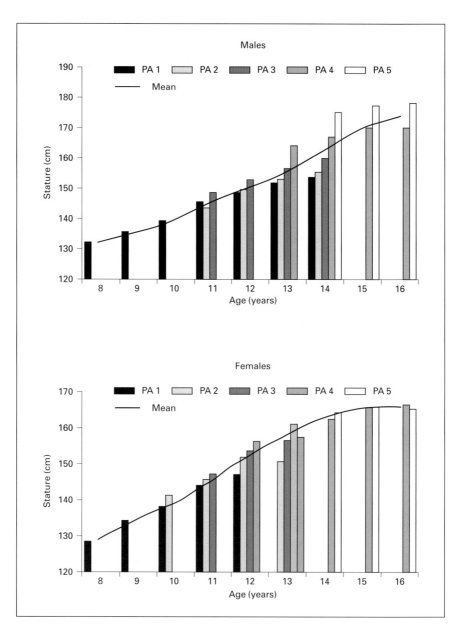

Fig. 1. Mean values for stature by age and stage of pubescent development.

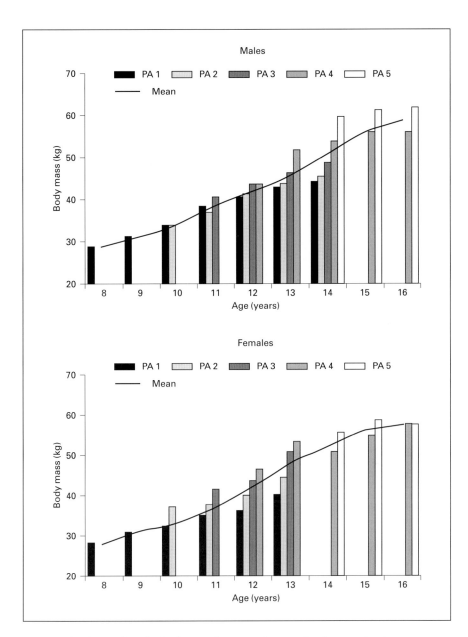

Fig. 2. Mean values for body mass by age and stage of pubescent development.

mately 14–15 years for males and at approximately 12–13 years for females. As for the stature results, those subjects who mature early are heavier than average. The later developers tend to be lighter than average at each of the ages beyond 12 years for boys and 10 years for girls. For example, at 13 years of age for the female sample, subjects who were still PA stage 2 were 7.7 kg lighter than average, while subjects who had reached PA stage 5 were 5.2 kg heavier than average.

Changes in adiposity with age for males and females are shown in figure 3. The average growth curve for males demonstrates a slight rise in the sum of five skinfolds up to age 12. This was predominantly due to the existence of a group of early maturers (PA stage 3) at 11 and 12 years (n = 20) with higher than average levels of body fat. As expected though, mean skinfold sum declined between 12 and 15 years as the majority of boys experienced their adolescent growth spurt. This phenomenon has been well documented [7].

The average growth curve for females demonstrates a steady increase in adiposity from 8 to 12 years, with a small plateau at 11–12 years. Those subjects who mature early have greater adiposity than average, while the later developers have lower levels of body fat than average at each of the ages beyond 10 years. For example, at 11 years of age, subjects who were still pre-adolescent had a Sum5SF 5.8 mm lower than average, while subjects who had reached PA stage 3 scored 14.8 mm greater than average. Similarly at 13 years, subjects who were still at PA stage 3 had a Sum5SF 12.9 mm lower than average, while subjects who had reached PA stage 5 scored 19.8 mm greater than average.

Gender Comparison: Pre-Adolescent

There has recently been a considerable increase in the amount of co-educational sport competition for young children. It is generally presumed by sport administrators that boys and girls can compete on equal terms in most activities until the onset of puberty, but there is a lack of scientific data to substantiate such a claim. The purpose of a study by Blanksby et al. [8] was to examine whether any differences existed between selected anatomical and physiological characteristics of pre-adolescent males and females. The results with respect to body composition are presented in table 1.

Subjects (n = 202) aged 7–12 years were rated by a medical practitioner as pre-adolescent according to the pubescence assessment standards for pubic hair [2]. A series of analyses of variance were performed to ascertain differences between males and females over each age and training group classification. In this analysis, a hierarchical approach was necessary so that any significant

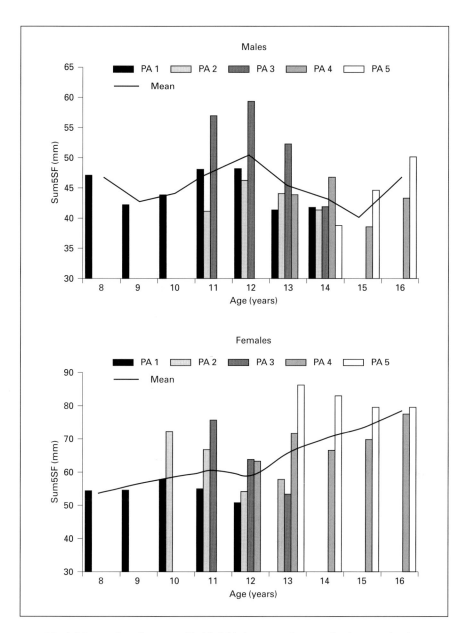

Fig. 3. Mean values for sum of 5 skinfolds by age and stage of pubescent development.

Table 1. Morphology characteristics of pre-adolescent males and females

Variable	F ratio	Gender difference
Stature	0.74	male = female
Body mass	0.20	male = female
Sum5SF	17.61*	male < female
Endomorphy	24.85*	male < female
Mesomorphy	9.20*	male > female
Ectomorphy	1.12	male = female

* $p < 0.025$.

age or training group effect could be accounted for prior to assessing the gender main effect. This procedure was employed due to the unbalanced nature of the research design.

Interactions between age, training group and gender were not significant which indicated that gender effects did not depend on training group or age. Therefore, interaction terms were dropped from the model and the data were then pooled. A significance level of 0.025 was adopted to compensate for the overall possibility of a type I error given the multiple F tests employed. Table 1 shows the comparison of male and female results for selected parameters.

Although some studies have shown pre-adolescent boys to be slightly larger than girls, the results of this study are in accord with the majority, in which no differences are noted for stature or body mass.

Conflicting evidence also exists within the literature relating to average levels of body fat in pre-adolescent boys and girls. The male subjects in this study had less body fat than the females. Sinclair [9] has stated that the fat content of the body decreased from 1 to 8 years of age, and that this decrease was less for girls than for boys. In contrast to this view, other researchers report that body fat differences between the sexes do not emerge until adolescence, at which time males experienced a decrease in subcutaneous fat, whereas females showed an increase.

A comparison of the somatotype components revealed that the mean endomorphy rating of the females was higher than that of the males. However, males demonstrated a significantly greater mesomorphy rating than the females. In contrast, there was no significant gender difference for the mean ectomorphy ratings. This study agrees with the findings of Malina and Rarick [10] that sex differences in body size are generally minor during the pre-adolescent years.

Table 2. Descriptive and ANOVA summary statistics for competitive swimmers (n = 37), tennis players (n = 61) and non-competitors (n = 104)

Variables	F ratio	Swimmers		Tennis players		Non-competitors	
		mean	range	mean	range	mean	range
Stature, cm	0.41	141.9	123.6–165.7	138.6	118.0–158.9	137.3	119.7–165.1
Body mass, kg	0.06	33.5	22.4–51.5	32.1	23.2–56.8	31.6	22.4–53.5
Sum3SF, mm	0.35	34.5	19.6–72.7	35.1	17.1–99.3	37.0	17.3–85.9
Endomorphy	0.47	2.6	1.5–5.5	2.6	1.0–6.5	2.8	1.0–5.5
Mesomorphy	0.53	4.0	2.2–5.5	4.1	2.5–6.0	4.0	2.0–6.5
Ectomorphy	0.52	3.8	1.0–6.0	3.5	1.0–6.0	3.4	0.5–6.0

Activity Group Comparisons: Pre-Adolescent

This mixed longitudinal study [11] sought to determine if there were any inherent anatomical and physiological differences between successful participants in competitive swimming and tennis, and a population of non-competitive children. A series of analyses of variance were applied using a hierarchical approach to the partitioning of the total sum of squares, due to the unbalanced nature of the research design [12].

For those variables where the main effect F ratio indicated a significant difference, paired t tests (one-tailed) were employed to determine those groups between which the significant differences ($p < 0.0167$) existed. Several F tests in the analysis proved to be non-significant. In order to avoid accepting a false null hypothesis (type II error), statistical power was calculated for each analysis of variance. It was assumed that the measures were normally distributed, with a common error variance. For all analyses, a statistical power greater than 0.8 was achieved with the sample size used in this study.

The means and ranges of scores of selected parameters for each group are presented in table 2. The mean pooled values are poor representations of the data since each group comprised children from 7 to 12 years. Therefore, a range of values was added to provide some indication of the spread of scores recorded from the sample.

The competitors did not differ from the non-competitors in stature, body mass or somatotype. Adiposity, as determined by the sum of three skinfold measures (triceps, subscapular, supra-iliac), was also similar for the three activity groups. This result was in contrast to that of earlier studies [13] that showed young swimmers to have lower than normal levels of fat deposition. A high percentage of body fat would be detrimental to both swimming and tennis performance. While a small amount of body fat could provide buoyancy advantages for the swimmer and added insulation if training in cold water, the detrimental effects of increased energy expenditure to move the added bulk and the increase in frontal resistance would appear to outweigh any advantage. The weight-supportive nature of tennis dictates that high levels of body fat would be contraindicated for success in this sport.

The results of this investigation clearly demonstrated that young, competitive children in swimming and tennis showed no body shape, composition or size differences at this stage of development when compared with non-competitors.

Activity Group Comparisons: Adolescent Swimmers

Studies of mature, elite swimmers have shown them to be superior to the average population in many physical capacities and physiological functions. It might therefore be assumed that differences occur between competitive swimmers and non-competitors in growth through adolescence or early post-adolescence. This study [14] sought to examine whether any changes occurred between competitors in intensive swimming training and non-competitors on selected physical and physiological characteristics through adolescence. If significant differences occurred, this could enable the identification of growth stages when the application of talent identification strategies may be possible.

Data for 95 competitive swimmers (38 male, 57 female) and 102 non-competitors (38 male, 64 female) were selected for this investigation. Data were employed only when the subject was last identified in PA stage 1, and when first identified as reaching successive PA stages 2–5. Because all subjects were not able to provide continuous data for each pubescent stage, a mixed longitudinal design was employed.

Sufficient evidence exists [15] to demonstrate that adolescent males differ from females in many morphological and physiological characteristics. Hence, it was pertinent to consider each gender separately in the data analysis. A series of two-factor analyses of variance were used to contrast swimmers and non-competitors at each pubescent stage. Where a significant F ratio ($p < 0.05$) for the treatment main effect was recorded, a Tukey's HSD post-hoc comparison was used to identify at which PA stage the groups were different.

Furthermore, several F tests in the analysis proved to be non-significant. In order to avoid accepting a false null hypothesis (type II error), statistical power was calculated for each analysis of variance, assuming that the measures were normally distributed, with a common error variance. For all analyses, a statistical power greater than 0.8 was achieved, given the sample size in this study.

Table 3. Mean scores for competitive swimmers and non-competitors by pubescent stage

Variable	Swimmers					Non-competitors				
	PA stage					PA stage				
	1	2	3	4	5	1	2	3	4	5
Males										
n	16	21	25	31	13	21	22	29	15	7
Age, months	146.2	149.7	156.2	169.0	187.0	144.1	146.0	152.2	161.7	183.6
Stature, cm	151.7	152.6	156.5	167.0	177.5	148.7	150.2	153.8	160.1	173.9
Body mass, kg	41.7	42.5	46.1	54.7	65.7	38.7	40.5	43.4	47.5	62.1
Sum5SF, mm	47.1	46.0	47.1	42.0	39.7	51.5	47.8	50.8	48.8	58.8
Endomorphy	2.6	2.5	2.5	2.4	2.1	2.8	2.9	2.9	2.5	2.9
Mesomorphy	4.4	4.2	4.4	4.3	4.4	4.0	4.0	4.1	4.0	4.2
Ectomorphy	3.5	3.6	3.5	3.7	3.7	3.7	3.6	3.6	3.9	3.6
Females										
n	19	29	34	51	31	32	37	45	45	23
Age, months	137.3	143.0	147.4	157.5	169.4	133.6	139.3	144.4	156.1	169.9
Stature, cm	144.2	147.4	152.5	158.8	162.9	145.2	148.6	152.2	159.8	162.7
Body mass, kg	34.9	37.9	41.1	48.6	55.8	36.2	39.6	42.0	48.7	56.1
Sum5SF, mm	46.0	53.2	49.8	57.4	53.3	53.6	59.0	47.9	52.8	62.0
Endomorphy	2.7	2.9	2.9	3.3	4.4	3.3	3.8	3.7	3.9	4.8
Mesomorphy	3.7	3.6	3.4	3.4	3.7	3.5	3.8	3.6	3.2	3.7
Ectomorphy	3.9	3.7	3.9	3.5	2.8	3.7	3.6	3.6	3.6	2.7

Descriptive statistics for male and female samples are presented in table 3. The following discussion will consider the ANOVA summary statistics in table 4 separately for males and females. As expected, a significant ($p < 0.05$) main effect F ratio was observed with increased maturation for most variables. However, the primary concern in the following discussion focuses on the activity group (ACT) main effect and the ACT × PA interactions.

Male Comparisons

The ACT group comparisons for body morphology variables show differences in body mass and stature at PA stage 4 only, with swimmers being larger than the non-competitors. This difference was not continued at PA stage 5 and might reflect the drop in sample size at this final level of maturation. In contrast, differences between the ACT groups in body composition were found only at PA stage 5. That is, despite the extra training load undertaken by the swimmers, no differences in subcutaneous fat levels were found for male adolescents up to PA stage 4. Thereafter, significantly lower total skinfold

Table 4. ANOVA summary and post-hoc comparisons for body morphology parameters

| Variable | Main effects F ratio | | | Post-hoc Tukeys HSD | | | | |
| | | | | PA stage | | | | |
	ACT	PA	ACT × PA	1	2	3	4	5
Males								
Age	3.12	42.19**	0.22	–	–	–	–	–
Stature	16.88**	79.47**	1.44	–	–	–	s > nc	–
Body mass	19.76**	77.10**	0.93	–	–	–	s > nc	–
Sum5SF	5.26*	0.42	0.95	–	–	–	–	s < nc
Endomorphy	4.65*	0.54	0.36	–	–	–	–	s < nc
Mesomorphy	7.04*	0.44	0.27	–	–	–	–	–
Ectomorphy	1.12	0.70	0.16	–	–	–	–	–
Females								
Age	3.26	82.80**	0.38	–	–	–	–	–
Stature	0.53	74.13**	0.21	–	–	–	–	–
Body mass	1.29	93.48**	0.19	–	–	–	–	–
Sum5SF	0.76	2.62	1.74	–	–	–	–	–
Endomorphy	26.60**	14.02**	0.29	–	s < nc	s < nc	s < nc	s < nc
Mesomorphy	0.16	2.02	0.83	–	–	–	–	–
Ectomorphy	0.46	7.41**	0.47	–	–	–	–	–

* $p < 0.05$, ** $p < 0.01$.

scores and endomorphy ratings were exhibited by the swimmers. This result is somewhat contrary to the findings of earlier studies [13] which showed young swimmers (13–15 years) to have lower than average levels of fat deposition. No differences were shown for mesomorphy or ectomorphy with male swimmers and tennis players.

Female Comparisons

The ACT group comparisons for body morphology variables show very few differences between female swimmers and non-competitors. Furthermore, no differences were recorded at the pre-adolescent stage of maturity. Results for the age variable confirm the findings of previous research [16] in which elite swimmers were similar or slightly advanced in maturity compared with the normal population. Similarly, no stature or body mass differences were recorded, a result which remains at variance with other studies on female swimmers [17].

A further inspection of table 4 provides seemingly conflicting results for the sum of skinfolds and endomorphy measures of body composition. While no significant ACT differences were recorded for the sum of skinfold scores, swimmers scored significantly lower on endomorphy from PA stage 2 when compared to non-competitors. This reinforces the need for standardised reporting of skinfold data and the use of a sufficient number of sites. Since the endomorphy variable is calculated from the sum of only three skinfold measurements in the upper body, it does not provide a completely representative sampling of subcutaneous fat deposition. No differences were reported for the mesomorphy or ectomorphy components of somatotype, which was similar to the result for males.

Discussion and Implications

For ease in the management of research, one might retrospectively compare the relationships between morphological and physiological parameters of elite performers with some control population. However, this study monitored structural changes over time among two, clearly identifiable activity groups. This form of research design provides a better chance of identifying those factors that discriminate talented performers from the general population, than data from retrospective studies.

This study has shown clearly that certain important measurements for successful swimming performance do not begin to discriminate the elite from control populations until during the later stages of pubescent development, while other differences occur after adolescence. It should be acknowledged that many of the variables that discriminate between talented individuals and non-competitors will respond to specific training from an early age. That is, variables such as muscular strength, body composition and exercise capacity possess both genetically determined and environmentally enhanced components. Thus, the type and severity of training prior to, and during, early adolescence will affect the utility of such measures for talent identification purposes. Nevertheless, such measures may still provide a meaningful comparison of swimmers, especially when used in combination with other physical features.

Activity Group Comparisons: Adolescent Tennis Players

One of the major problems that faces the sports scientist, whether working with national level performers or with promising juniors, is to identify precisely those variables that differentiate the elite player from those of lesser ability in the playing population. The identification of specific variables that correlate highly with tennis performance assists in the development of talented persons who can be coached to maximise their inherent genotypic, and developed phenotypic, traits in achieving tennis playing success.

This section examines the relationship between playing success and selected morphological variables collected during a longitudinal study of junior tennis players and matched controls. By following the tennis players' performances prospectively, this study [19] is unique in its attempt to observe the stability of selected discriminatory factors through the adolescent period. The aim was to determine whether certain traits are important in discriminating tennis performance through adolescence.

Tennis players (10–12 years) who regularly attained a semifinal position in the Western Australian Lawn Tennis Association sanctioned tournaments formed tennis group A (TA), while players who occasionally attained a quarter final position in these tournaments were classified as tennis group B (TB). A similar number of non-competitive controls (C) were matched at the 11-years age classification on height and body mass with the subjects from the two tennis groups.

A series of two-factor analyses of variance was used to contrast TA, TB and C groups. As no significant interaction was found within the analysis for any variable, tests for simple main effects were considered appropriate [18]. Where a significant F ratio (p<0.05) for the treatment main effect was recorded, a Scheffe post-hoc comparison was used to identify which activity groups were different.

Descriptive statistics for the male and female samples are presented in table 5, and summary results for the two-factor ANOVA and post-hoc Scheffe tests are contained within table 6. While many variables predictably demonstrate a significant growth with increasing age, the primary concern of this paper is focussed on activity group differences. Thus the discussion will be biased towards the activity group main effect and group × age interactions, with each gender treated separately.

Male Comparisons
The group comparisons for physical variables (table 6) show no differences in stature or body mass. After matching for these parameters at age 11 years, the groups remained similar through to 15 years of age. However, in terms of body composition and body type, a significant difference between groups was identified. At each age category, TA possessed lower levels of body fat than the controls. Players in TB were situated between these extreme groups and, therefore, did not significantly differ from either. A clear stratum of body fat levels has been identified such that the higher ranked players are leaner than the lower ranked players, followed by the controls. This characteristic remains stable through the 11- to 15-year age range, and would appear to be due to the greater work output and energy expenditure in the training level of players in TA.

Table 5. Mean scores for competitive tennis players and non-competitors by age group

Variable	Tennis A			Tennis B			Controls		
	11 years	13 years	15 years	11 years	13 years	15 years	11 years	13 years	15 years
Males									
n	17	27	13	23	27	11	25	31	11
Stature, cm	142.4	153.4	169.6	143.7	152.7	162.0	143.4	154.9	168.6
Body mass, kg	33.5	41.1	54.0	35.6	41.8	50.9	35.6	44.5	55.2
Sum5SF, mm	39.9	42.0	36.2	45.7	47.0	39.4	50.2	53.9	47.7
Endomorphy	2.2	2.2	1.9	2.5	2.5	2.1	2.7	2.9	2.3
Mesomorphy	4.0	3.9	3.9	4.1	4.1	4.5	4.2	4.2	4.0
Ectomorphy	3.8	4.1	4.5	3.5	3.8	3.4	3.4	3.6	4.0
Females									
n	13	16	15	19	23	11	23	29	17
Stature, cm	145.1	159.0	161.5	141.5	152.9	161.1	146.1	157.8	166.2
Body mass, kg	36.4	44.9	54.2	35.2	44.8	55.7	37.5	46.4	56.2
Sum5SF, mm	57.4	52.2	65.7	54.5	66.7	91.4	65.2	66.8	79.6
Endomorphy	3.4	2.9	3.9	3.2	3.7	5.0	3.8	3.7	4.7
Mesomorphy	3.7	2.9	3.2	3.9	4.0	4.2	3.6	3.2	3.3
Ectomorphy	3.7	4.3	3.4	3.2	3.2	2.4	3.4	3.9	3.3

Despite the similarity between groups in terms of height and mass, group TA was significantly more linear in body type than the control group as shown by the ectomorphy values. For males, the ecto-mesomorphic body type would appear to be a required characteristic for successful tennis performance at the professional level [20] and presumably the linearity component may be a discriminatory factor from the early ages tested in this study.

Female Comparisons

The group comparisons for physical variables (table 6) show that for females, as for males, height and mass were not discriminating factors for tennis performance. Players in TB were smaller than the other sub-samples but the C and TA groups did not differ. However, as with the males, body composition was an important indicator of tennis performance for 11- to 15-year-old females. Players in TA were leaner than the control group as demonstrated in the endomorphy and Sum5SF scores. The players in TB once again were placed between these extreme groups (table 6). Although significant differences were recorded between the groups on the mesomorphy and ecto-morphy components, no clear effects on performance could be elicited from these results. Players in TA, together with the control group, were more ecto-

Table 6. ANOVA summary and post-hoc comparisons for body morphology parameters

Variable	Main effects F ratio			Post-hoc Scheffe		
	Gp	age	Gp × age	TA vs. TB	TA vs. C	TB vs. C
Males						
Stature	2.60	137.00*	1.90	–	–	–
Body mass	2.15	85.82*	0.77	–	–	–
Sum5SF	5.00*	1.54	0.05	TA = TB	TA < C	TB = C
Endomorphy	3.99*	2.33	0.09	TA = TB	TA < C	TB = C
Mesomorphy	1.18	0.03	0.58	–	–	–
Ectomorphy	3.70*	1.40	0.64	TA = TB	TA > C	TB = C
Females						
Stature	8.74*	113.28*	0.32	TA > TB	TA = C	TB < C
Body Mass	0.82	77.06*	0.12	–	–	–
Sum5SF	3.25*	7.19*	1.16	TA = TB	TA < C	TB = C
Endomorphy	3.36*	9.46*	0.99	TA = TB	TA < C	TB = C
Mesomorphy	10.97*	2.81	1.28	TA > TB	TA = C	TB = C
Ectomorphy	7.14*	5.01*	0.50	TA > TB	TA = C	TB < C

* Significant at $p < 0.05$.

morphic and less mesomorphic than the players in TB. Copley [20] had shown that professional female players were more endo-mesomorphic than amateur players who tended to be more ecto-mesomorphic.

Conclusion

To the authors' knowledge this was the first time that subjects were selected for a longitudinal study on the basis of sporting success at an early age. In earlier studies, the subjects had been measured and then divided into sub-groups before the data were analysed. The sports of swimming and tennis were chosen for this study because of their co-educational nature, their popularity, the availability of high-level competitors, and because of the bilateral and horizontal nature of swimming versus the on-land, unilateral nature of tennis.

Not only was a successful retention of a high quality, mixed longitudinal sample achieved over the 5-year duration of the project, but the inclusion of pubescence assessment within the test battery added a unique dimension to the research. Thus, a stratification of the sample according to biological age for a number of the analyses was possible, which is a critical variable when attempting to tease out subtle group differences during the highly variable phase of growth through adolescence. Further work in this area is encouraged to more accurately delineate elements of successful performance which maximise their sporting opportunities.

References

1   Blanksby BA, Bloomfield J, Ackland TR, Elliott BC, Morton AR: Athletics, Growth and Development in Children. Chur, Harwood Academic Press, 1994.
2   Tanner JM: Growth at Adolescence, ed 2. Oxford, Blackwell Scientific Publications, 1962.
3   Montague AMF: A Handbook of Anthropometry. Springfield, Thomas, 1960.
4   Hrdlicka A: Practical Anthropometry, ed 3. Philadelphia, Wistar Institute, 1947.
5   Norton K, Whittingham N, Carter JEL, Kerr D, Gore C, Marfell-Jones M: Measurement techniques in anthropometry; in Norton K, Olds T (eds): Anthropometrica. Sydney, UNSW Press, 1996.
6   Carter JEL: The Heath-Carter Somatotype Method. San Diego, San Diego State University Press, 1980.
7   Forbes G: Body composition in adolescence; in Falkner F, Tanner JM (eds): Human Growth, vol 2. London, Baillière Tindall Paul, 1978.
8   Blanksby BA, Bloomfield J, Elliott BC, Ackland TR, Morton AR: The anatomical and physiological characteristics of pre-adolescent males and females. Aust Paediatr J 1986;22:177–180.
9   Sinclair D: Human Growth after Birth, ed 3. London, Oxford University Press, 1978.
10 Malina RM, Rarick GL: Growth, physique and motor performance; in Rarick GL (ed): Physical Activity: Human Growth and Development. New York, Academic Press, 1973.
11 Bloomfield J, Blanksby BA, Ackland TR, Elliott BC: The anatomical and physiological characteristics of preadolescent swimmers, tennis players and non-competitors. Aust J Sci Med Sport 1985; 17:19–23.
12 Aitken M: The analysis of unbalanced cross-classifications. J Royal Statist Soc [A] 1978;141:195–222.
13 Vaccaro P, Vaccaro P, Clarke DH, Morris AF: Physiological characteristics of young well-trained swimmers. Eur J Appl Physiol 1980;44:61–66.
14 Bloomfield J, Blanksby BA, Ackland TR: Morphological and physiological growth of competitive swimmers and non-competitors through adolescence. Aust J Sci Med Sport 1990;22:4–12.
15 Marshall WA: Puberty; in Falkner F, Tanner JM (eds): Human Growth, vol 2. London, Baillière Tindall Paul, 1978.
16 Malina RM: Menarche in athletes: A synthesis and hypothesis. Ann Hum Biol 1983;10:1–24.
17 Andrew GM, Becklake MR, Guleria JS, Bates DV: Heart and lung functions in swimmers and non-athletes during growth. J Appl Physiol 1972;32:245–251.
18 Winer BJ: Statistical Principles in Experimental Design, ed 2. New York, McGraw-Hill, 1971.
19 Elliott BC, Ackland TR, Blanksby BA, Bloomfield J: A prospective study of the physiological and kinanthropometric indicators of junior tennis performance. Aust J Sci Med Sport 1990;22:87–92.
20 Copley BB: A morphological and physiological study of tennis players with special reference to the effects of training. South Afr J Sports Phys Educ Recr 980;3:33–44.

Assoc. Prof. Tim Ackland, Department of Human Movement and Exercise Science,
The University of Western Australia, Nedlands WA 6907 (Australia)
Tel. +61 8 9380 2668, Fax +61 9 9380 1039, E-Mail tackland@cyllene.uwa.edu.au

Jürimäe T, Hills AP (eds): Body Composition Assessment in Children and Adolescents.
Med Sport Sci. Basel, Karger, 2001, vol 44, pp 132–138

....

Explaining Cardiovascular Disease Risk Factor Variability in Obese Teenagers Using Measured and Predicted Values of Visceral Adipose Tissue

Scott Owens, Mark Litaker, Bernard Gutin

Georgia Prevention Institute, Department of Pediatrics, Medical College of Georgia, Augusta, Ga., USA

Recent studies in obese young people have shown that visceral adipose tissue (VAT) tends to explain greater proportions of the variance in cardiovascular disease (CVD) risk factors than do other measures of adiposity such as total percent body fat, total body fat mass, waist-to-hip ratio or subcutaneous abdominal adipose tissue [1–3]. VAT measurements are derived from MRI or CT scans and tend to be reported in one of two ways: (1) as a surface area in cm^2 from a single transverse slice at the approximate level of the umbilicus (4th lumbar vertebra, L4), or (2) as a volume measurement in cm^3 (or liters) from a series of 5–7 transverse slices from the abdominal region [4–6]. The single-slice method is less time consuming, appears to facilitate comparisons between studies, and, in the case of CT, exposes subjects to a lower radiation dose. Multi-slice values are perhaps more satisfying statistically since they provide information from a larger segment of the abdominal region and potentially provide for a more stable measure. Adult studies have reported single- and multi-slice measures of VAT to be highly correlated [4, 7], although a study that reported on the relationships between single- and multi-slice measures of VAT and CVD risk factors found the multi-slice measure to be more strongly associated with the risk factors [5]. Little is known about the nature of these relationships in youths.

A third type of VAT data comes from VAT prediction equations based on simple anthropometric measures. This method would obviate the need for access to expensive MRI or CT technology. To date, the explanatory power of predicted VAT relative to CVD risk factors is unknown. In the present study, we compare three approaches, that is, single-slice, multi-slice, and VAT predicted from simple anthropometric indices, in terms of their power to explain the variability in CVD risk factors in a group of obese teenagers.

Methods

Subjects were 80 apparently healthy, sedentary (as per self-report), obese teenagers (26 boys, 54 girls) 13–16 years of age. Recruitment was accomplished with promotional flyers distributed through selected public and private schools in Augusta, Georgia. To be included in the study, a child needed to have a triceps skinfold greater than the 85th percentile for gender, age and ethnicity [8]. Ethnicity was by self-designation of the parent. Tanner stage was not determined, but all girls reported having achieved menarche. Interested parents and teenagers attended an orientation session and both gave informed consent in accordance with procedures of our Human Assurance Committee.

VAT Measures

VAT was determined in the Department of Radiology at the Medical College of Georgia utilizing a 1.5-Tesla MRI system (General Electric Medical Systems, Milwaukee, Wisc., USA). Spin echo techniques were used to produce T1 weighted images demonstrating good contrast between adipose and non-adipose tissues [4]. Details of the MRI acquisition were as follows: repetition time: 450 ms; echo time: 12 ms; field of view: 400–480 mm; matrix: 192×256; number of excitations: 1. Respiratory compensation was used to reduce artifacts caused by respiratory motion. With subjects in the supine position, a series of five, 1-cm-thick, transverse images was acquired beginning at the inferior border of the fifth lumbar vertebra and proceeding towards the head. A 2-mm gap between images was utilized to prevent cross-talk. Tissues superior to and inferior to the five slices were saturated to prevent blood flow in the aorta or inferior vena cava from appearing as high intensity artifacts in the images. VAT was segmented by thresholding and quantified as adipose tissue within a region of interest bounded by the innermost aspect of the abdominal and oblique muscle walls and the posterior aspect of the vertebral body. The single-slice value for VAT was obtained from the L4–L5 space and is reported in terms of surface area (cm^2). The multi-slice VAT measurement is reported in cm^3 and was derived by multiplying the surface area for the individual images by the image width (1 cm) and then summing across the five images. To reduce inter-observer variability, all images were analyzed by the same experienced observer. The intra-class correlation coefficients for VAT from separate-day repeat analyses of the same scans exceeded 0.99.

To obtain a predicted value for VAT, we utilized an equation previously developed in the author's laboratory for predicting VAT at L4 (cm^2) based on simple anthropometric measurements obtained from 76 Black and White obese youths aged 7–16 years [9]. Specifically, the VAT prediction equation is:

$$-124.06 + 16.67 \text{ (ethnicity)} + 4.15 \text{ (sagittal diameter)} + 100.89 \text{ (waist-to-hip ratio)},$$

where ethnicity is coded as 0 = Black and 1 = White.

Table 1. Descriptive characteristics of subjects (n = 80)

Variable	Mean	SD
Age, years	14.9	1.3
Height, cm	164.9	7.3
Weight kg	95.0	19.5
VAT: L4 single slice, cm^2	61.4	27.3
VAT: multi-slice, cm^3	300.7	125.9
VAT: L4 predicted, cm^2	67.6	20.1

Blood Parameters

For blood sampling, subjects reported to the laboratory between 8 and 9 a.m. following a 12-hour fast. A 20-ml blood sample was obtained from an antecubital vein into vacutainers containing EDTA. Duplicate samples were analyzed for triglycerides, total cholesterol, high-density lipoprotein cholesterol (HDLC), low-density lipoprotein cholesterol (LDLC), apo-lipoprotein B (Apo B), and insulin at the Emory Lipid Research Laboratory which is certified by the College of American Pathologists and participates in the National Heart, Lung and Blood/Centers for Disease Control Lipid Standardization Program.

Resting Blood Pressure

Resting blood pressure measured with an automated BP monitor (Dinamap, Critikon, Inc., Tampa, Fla., USA). Measurements were obtained after 10 min of rest in the supine position with an appropriately sized cuff placed on the left arm. Five readings were taken at one minute intervals and the last three were averaged. In keeping with our current research interests and the desire to limit the number of variables reported here, we present data for systolic blood pressure only.

Data Analysis

Data were examined first for deviations from normality. As no significant deviations were found, Pearson correlations were determined between single-slice, multi-slice, and predicted VAT. Simple linear regression was used to determine the proportion of variance explained by the respective VAT measures for each of the CVD risk factors. Multiple linear regression was used to evaluate whether including predicted VAT and multi-slice VAT (or single VAT) in the same model resulted in either variable explaining significant proportions of the variance beyond that explained by the other variable.

Results

Table 1 shows the descriptive statistics for the 80 subjects. Table 2 displays mean values for the CVD risk factors for the combined 80 subjects. The simple correlations between the three measures of VAT are shown in table 3. The

Table 2. Mean values for cardiovascular risk factors
(n = 80)

Variable	Mean	SD
Triglycerides, mg/dl	93.1	60.7
Total cholesterol, mg/dl	164.6	34.2
HDL cholesterol, mg/dl	42.3	9.5
Total cholesterol/HDLC	4.1	1.2
LDL cholesterol, mg/dl	108.1	30.5
Apo B, mg/dl	73.3	18.8
Insulin, μU/l	24.5	13.6
Systolic blood pressure, mm Hg	112.2	14.5

Table 3. Correlations* among three measures of VAT

Variable	L4 single-slice	Multi-slice	L4 predicted
L4 single-slice	–	0.98	0.77
Multi-slice	0.98	–	0.76

* p values for all correlations were <0.001.

VAT measures were all highly correlated (p < 0.001), especially the single- and multi-slice measures. Table 4 displays the proportions of variance explained by each of the three VAT measures for each of the CVD risk factors. The single-slice and multi-slice VAT explained nearly identical proportions of the variance in each of the seven CVD risk factors examined. The multiple linear regressions indicated that predicted VAT explained a significant proportion of variance not explained by single-slice VAT (p = 0.013) or by multi-slice VAT (p = 0.007) only in the case of insulin. Table 5 shows the proportions of variance explained for the CVD risk factors by the three individual variables from the VAT prediction equation.

Discussion

This appears to be the first study to examine single-slice, multi-slice, and predicted VAT in terms of their explanatory power for CVD risk factors. We found that single-slice and multi-slice VAT explained nearly identical propor-

Table 4. Proportion of variance in CVD risk factors explained (R^2) by VAT measures

Dependent variable	VAT L4 single-slice R^2	VAT multi-slice R^2	VAT L4 predicted R^2
Triglycerides	0.08	0.09	0.12
Total cholesterol	0.08	0.08	0.10
HDL cholesterol	0.06	0.06	0.06
Total cholesterol/HDLC	0.18	0.18	0.16
LDL cholesterol	0.07	0.08	0.09
Apo B	0.14	0.16	0.16
Insulin	0.06	0.05	0.13*
Systolic blood pressure	0.10	0.12	0.14

* In multiple linear regression, predicted VAT explained a significant proportion of variance not explained by single-slice VAT ($p = 0.013$) or by multi-slice VAT ($p = 0.007$).

Table 5. Proportion of variance in CVD risk factors explained (R^2) by individual components of the VAT prediction equation

Dependent variable	Ethnicity R^2	Sagittal diameter R^2	Waist-to-hip ratio R^2
Triglycerides	0.15	0.04	0.03
Total cholesterol	0.00	0.04	0.18
HDL cholesterol	0.10	0.01	0.02
Total cholesterol/HDLC	0.06	0.04	0.16
LDL cholesterol	0.00	0.04	0.18
Apo B	0.04	0.05	0.18
Insulin	0.00	0.16	0.06
Systolic blood pressure	0.00	0.13	0.08

tions of the variance in each of the seven CVD risk factors examined. In a study of obese men, Rissanen et al. [5] reported multi-slice VAT explained somewhat greater proportions of the variance than did single-slice VAT for triglycerides ($r^2 = 0.50$, $p < 0.01$ vs. $r^2 = 0.29$, $p < 0.05$) and Apo B/LDLC ($r^2 = 0.50$, $p < 0.01$ vs. $r^2 = 0.36$, $p < 0.05$). The authors concluded, nevertheless, that the two VAT measures were similar enough in their association with the risk factors that either could be used. The finding that the differences between single- and multi-slice measures were even less than observed by Rissanen et al. [5] supports the notion of the virtual interchangeability of the two VAT measures, at least in cross-sectional studies. Some authors have suggested that in intervention studies where changes in VAT are examined over time, there may be reason to favor the multi-slice approach. For example, in their study of the effects of energy restriction and exercise on VAT, Ross and Rissanen noted a trend suggesting that VAT from the upper abdomen was greater than from the lower abdomen, indicating that observations regarding changes in VAT may be influenced by the region of the abdomen that is studied [10]. This scenario highlights the advantage of using a multi-slice model.

Interestingly, predicted VAT in the current study explained as much or more of the variability in six of the seven risk factors as did the directly measured VAT. Only in the case of insulin, however, did predicted VAT explain significant additional proportions of variance not explained by single- or multi-slice VAT. Recall that the VAT prediction equation included ethnicity, sagittal diameter, and waist-to-hip ratio. Table 5 shows the variance in the CVD risk factors explained by the individual components of the VAT prediction equation. Ethnicity was most strongly associated with triglycerides, whereas sagittal diameter was most strongly associated with insulin and systolic blood pressure. The waist-to-hip ratio was a relatively strong predictor of total cholesterol, total cholesterol/HDLC, LDLC, and Apo B. Thus, for five of the seven risk factors, one of the three variables from the VAT prediction equation explained more of the variance than did either the single-slice or multi-slice VAT measure. Hence, even though VAT has some explanatory power for CVD risk factors, other factors such as ethnicity, sagittal diameter, and waist-to-hip ratio can provide additional information. In the cases of triglycerides and HDL cholesterol, a multiple regression including both multi-slice VAT and ethnicity explained slightly more variability (compare with tables 3 and 4) than either variable individually ($R^2 = 0.18$ for triglycerides, $R^2 = 0.12$ for HDL-cholesterol). Including both waist-to-hip ratio and multi-slice VAT in multiple regression equations increased the variance explained in four of the lipid/lipoproteins ($R^2 = 0.19$ for total cholesterol, $R^2 = 0.22$ for total cholesterol/HDLC, $R^2 = 0.19$ for LDLC, $R^2 = 0.23$ for Apo B). With multi-slice VAT and sagittal diameter included, variance explained for systolic blood pressure was $R^2 = 0.16$.

The results of the current study confirm the findings of adult studies that show single- and multi-slice VAT are highly correlated, and that multi-VAT measures explain slightly more (up to 2% in our data) of the variance in CVD risk factors. The present data also suggest that a combination of simple anthropometric measures such as ethnicity, sagittal diameter, and waist-to-hip ratio can provide information about the variability in CVD risk factors in addition to that provided by VAT. Finally, it should be understood that while the current study was of a group of obese teenagers, findings from subjects who cover the entire range of fatness might differ from those discussed here.

Acknowledgment

This research was supported by a grant from the National Heart, Lung, and Blood Institute (HL55564).

References

1   Owens S, Gutin B, Ferguson M, Allison J, Karp W, Le N-A: Visceral adipose tissue and cardiovascular risk factors in obese children. J Pediatr 1998;133:41–45.
2   Brambilla P, Manzoni P, Sironi S, Simone P, Del Maschio A, di Natale B, Chiumello G: Peripheral and abdominal adiposity in childhood obesity. Int J Obes 1994;18:795–800.
3   Caprio S, Hyman LD, McCarthy S, Lange R, Bronson M, Tamborlane WV: Fat distribution and cardiovascular risk factors in obese adolescent girls: Importance of the intrabdominal fat depot. Am J Clin Nutr 1996;64:12–17.
4   Ross R, Leger L, Morris D, de Guise J, Guardo R: Quantification of adipose tissue by MRI: relationship with anthropometric variables. J Appl Physiol 1992;72:787–795.
5   Rissanen J, Hudson R, Ross R: Visceral adiposity, androgens, and plasma lipids in obese men. Metabolism 1994;43:1318–1323.
6   Owens S, Gutin B, Allison J, Riggs S, Ferguson M, Litaker M, Thompson W: Effect of physical training on total and visceral fat in obese children. Med Sci Sport Exerc 1999;31:143–148.
7   Kvist H, Chowdhury B, Grangard U, Tylen U, Sjostrom L: Total and visceral adipose-tissue volumes derived from measurements with computed tomography in adult men and women: Predictive equations. Am J Clin Nutr 1988;48:1351–1361.
8   Must A, Dallal GE, Dietz WH: Reference data for obesity: 85th and 95th percentiles of body mass index (wt/ht^2) and triceps skinfold thickness. Am J Clin Nutr 1991;53:839–846.
9   Owens S, Litaker M, Allison J, Riggs S, Ferguson M, Gutin B: Prediction of visceral adipose tissue from simple anthropometric measurements in youths with obesity. Obes Res 1999;7:16–22.
10 Ross R, Rissanen J: Mobilization of visceral and subcutaneous adipose tissue in response to energy restriction and exercise. Am J Clin Nutr 1994;60:695–703.

Scott Owens, PhD, Reid Gymnasium, Western Carolina University,
Cullowhee, NC 28723 (USA)
Tel. +1 (828) 293–3546, Fax +1 (828)-293–7645, E-Mail sgowens@wcu.edu

Jürimäe T, Hills AP (eds): Body Composition Assessment in Children and Adolescents.
Med Sport Sci. Basel, Karger, 2001, vol 44, pp 139–154

....

The Use of Different Prediction
Equations for the Assessment of Body
Composition in Young Female Gymnasts
– Is There a Best Equation?

A.L. Claessens, W. Delbroek, J. Lefevre

Department of Sports and Movement Sciences, Katholieke Universiteit Leuven,
Belgium

During the recent decades the number of children and youth involved in
organized, competitive sports has increased. As a consequence, youth sports
in general, and more specifically, elite sports for teenage youth are presently
a public phenomenon [1, 2]. Changes in expectations of performance at top
levels, together with the extreme training demands and the controlling of
young athletes by their coaches, parents, and the peer environment, has resulted
in public and medical concerns [2]. The prerequisites of athletic success in
many sports rely to a great extent upon physical characteristics, including
anthropometric dimensions, somatotype, and body composition [2–4]. The
relevance of morphology is especially evident in 'artistic' sports, such as ballet,
gymnastics, figure skating, and diving, wherein the body is a primary element
in obtaining high performance scores, and scoring may be influenced by the
perceptions of the judges [4–6]. The importance of a well-suited 'gymnastic-
specific' body build for reaching the highest level in artistic gymnastics is
well documented [7]. On average, compared to reference peers of the same
chronological age, top-level female gymnasts are characterized by a short
stature, light body mass, narrow hips with relatively broad shoulders, an ecto-
mesomorphic somatotype, a low percentage of body fat with a high fat-free
mass, and later maturation [7]. Gymnastic training commences at a very young
age – for example, in a representative sample of world-ranking female gymnasts
starting age was about 7.5 years [8]. In many teenage girls there is a latent
pressure to obtain the 'ideal' gymnastic-specific body build, especially to keep

their weight, and more specifically their percentage of body fat, as low as possible. This can lead to substantive physical and psychological problems [9, 10]. From a medical, health, and gymnastic-technical perspective, it is important to estimate body composition characteristics in these young athletes as accurately as possible. A variety of valid and reliable methods are available for estimating body composition in children and adolescents. For example, techniques include densitometry, hydrometry, body potassium, neutron activation analysis, and creatine excretion [11]. More recent sophisticated technologies, such as magnetic resonance imaging, computerized tomography scanning, and dual-energy X-ray absorptiometry have been developed [11]. Although all of these methods have been utilized for estimating body composition of children and adolescents, they are largely limited to the clinical or laboratory settings. Methods which can easily be applied in field testing are anthropometry, especially skinfolds, and bioelectrical impedance analysis (BIA) [12]. Several skinfold and BIA equations have been developed for use in the paediatric population [11, 12]. Questions arise as to which of these equations are 'valid' and appropriate for use in the gymnastic setting by trainers and/or coaches. In other words, is there some evidence, from a gymnastics point of view, that one equation is more of value than others?

The aim of this study therefore was to compare several skinfold and BIA equations for the estimation of body composition in the paediatric population in a group of young female gymnasts, and to 'validate' them against some 'external' criteria which are of relevance in the specific gymnastic setting.

Methods

Subjects

The sample consisted of 84 competitive and recreational female gymnasts from two prominent clubs in the Antwerp region in Flanders, Belgium. In these clubs, gymnasts are instructed from a beginners' level to national and international competitions. The mean age of the total group of gymnasts was 10.5 ± 2.6 years. The study was approved by the Medical Ethics Committee of the Faculty of Physical Education & Physiotherapy of the Katholieke Universiteit Leuven. Informed consent was given by the parents of all children involved in this study.

Tests and Variables

All gymnasts were investigated under standardized conditions in the laboratory setting on a battery of anthropometric and body composition measures, and physical fitness and gymnastic-specific performance tests. All measurements and tests were taken during one occasion and took approximately half a day.

Anthropometry. A battery of 26 anthropometric measures was taken: body mass; 7 length dimensions (stature, sitting height, acromial height, radial height, dactylion height,

Table 1. BIA and skinfold prediction equations used for the assessment of body composition in young female gymnasts

For-mula No.	Formula	Ref.
BIA formulae		
1	% fat = -8.4773+(0.4296 * BS)+(1.3405 * CG) -(0.845 * BIA index)+(0.3833 * W)	[14]
2	FFM = (2580 * BIA index)+(0.375 * W)+(10.5 * S) -(0.164 * AGE)-6.5	[15]
3	FFM = (0.633 * BIA index)+(0.274 * W) + (0.124 * REA)-8.583	[16]
4	FFM = (0.83 * BIA index)+4.43	[17]
Skinfold formulae		
5	% fat = (0.61 * Σ2)+5.1	[18]
6	% fat = 1.0987-(0.00122 * Σ3) +(0.00000263 * (Σ3)²)	[19]

BS = Biceps skinfold (mm); CG = calf girth (cm); BIA index = stature²/R; W = weight (kg); S = stature (cm); AGE = chronological age (years); REA = reactance (Ω); Σ2 = triceps + calf skinfolds (mm); Σ3 = triceps + subscapular + suprailiac skinfolds (mm).

tibial height, forearm length); 4 breadth dimensions (biacromial and biiliac diameters, humerus and femur widths); 8 circumferences (upper-arm flexed and relaxed, forearm, waist, hip, upper thigh, lower thigh, calf); and 6 skinfolds (biceps, triceps, subscapular, suprailiac, medial calf, front thigh). All bilateral measurements were taken on the left side of the body. Skinfolds were measured twice with a Harpenden skinfold caliper. When a difference between the two trials was more than 10%, a third trial was taken. For each skinfold, the mean of all trials was taken as the final measurement. All measurements were taken by well-trained anthropometrists assisted by a recorder who was familiar with the specific procedures. All observers were trained by one of the authors who is a criterion anthropometrist recognized by the International Society for the Advancement of Kinanthropometry (ISAK). For the description of the measurement techniques the reader is referred to Claessens et al. [12]. Only those measurements which are of relevance in this study (for calculating the body composition estimates) were selected and used for further analyses.

Body Composition Assessment by BIA. Resistance (Ω) and reactance (Ω) were measured by the bioelectrical impedance analyzer BIA 109 (Akern, Florence, Italy) according to the recommendations of the National Institute of Health Technology [13]. Fat-free mass (FFM) or percentage of body fat (% fat) were calculated according to different formulae which were

Table 2. Descriptive statistics for anthropometric and body composition characteristics in female gymnasts (n = 84)

Variable	Mean	SD
Anthropometry		
Body weight, kg	32.2	9.9
Stature, cm	138.9	13.7
Triceps skinfold, mm	9.6	2.5
Biceps skinfold, mm	4.6	1.5
Subscapular skinfold, mm	5.5	1.4
Suprailiac skinfold, mm	5.7	2.7
Calf skinfold, mm	9.8	3.2
Thigh skinfold, mm	14.0	3.6
Body composition		
Sum 6 skinfolds, mm	49.3	13.5
Resistance, Ω	704.1	82.6
% Fat		
Guo (No. 1)	18.8	3.0
Deurenberg (No. 2)	19.2	6.9
Houtkooper (No. 3)	15.7	3.9
Houtkooper (No. 4)	14.6	4.8
Slaughter (No. 5)	16.9	3.3
Thorland (No. 6)	11.1	2.6
Fat mass, kg		
Guo (No. 1)	6.3	2.7
Deurenberg (No. 2)	6.6	3.2
Houtkooper (No. 3)	5.3	2.7
Houtkooper (No. 4)	5.0	2.8
Slaughter (No. 5)	5.5	2.7
Thorland (No. 6)	3.7	2.0
Fat-free mass, kg		
Guo (No. 1)	26.5	7.6
Deurenberg (No. 2)	26.2	3.6
Houtkooper (No. 3)	27.4	7.6
Houtkooper (No. 4)	27.7	7.7
Slaughter (No. 5)	26.6	7.7
Thorland (No. 6)	28.5	8.2

specifically developed for the female paediatric population, and which could be applied to our study group. An overview of the formulae used, together with the necessary independent variables, is given in table 1.

Body Composition Assessment by Skinfold Equations. After reviewing the literature, two anthropometric equations for the estimation of percentage of body fat (% fat), were ascer-

Table 3. Descriptive characteristics for fitness and performance tests in female gymnasts (n = 84)

Variable	Mean	SD
Eurofit Test battery		
Flamingo Balance, n	10.1	6.5
Plate Tapping, s	15.3	3.7
Sit and Reach, cm	31.4	4.9
Standing Broad Jump, cm	167.0	27.0
Handgrip, kg	19.3	8.0
Sit-ups, n	27.1	7.3
Bent Arm Hang, s	29.2	19.6
Shuttle Run, s	21.3	1.5
Gymnastic-specific tests		
Strength shoulder flexion, kg	21.2	7.8
Strength shoulder extension, kg	28.9	12.3
Strength hip flexion, kg	20.0	7.9
Strength hip extension, kg	47.3	16.5
Flexible shoulders antep., °	32.9	22.0
Flexible shoulders retrop., °	86.7	13.7
Flexible hip flexion, °	75.2	14.6
Flexible hip extension, °	38.8	10.5

tained to be valid and applicable for use with subjects in this study, namely the equation developed by Slaughter et al. [18] and by Thorland et al. [19]. Both equations are illustrated in table 1.

Performance Tests. The performance of the gymnasts was tested in two ways: (1) in order to test the general physical fitness the Eurofit Test Battery was administered; (2) gymnastic-specific strength and flexibility tests were developed.

(1) *Eurofit Test Battery.* This test battery provides relevant information on an individual's basic motor abilities and consists of the following tests: Flamingo Balance (FB) – measuring total body balance; Plate Tapping (PT) – measuring speed of limb movement; Sit and Reach (SR) – measuring flexibility; Standing Broad Jump (SBJ) – measuring explosive strength; Handgrip (HG) – measuring static strength; Sit-ups (SU) – measuring trunk strength; Bent Arm Hang (BAH) – measuring functional strength; and Shuttle Run 10 × 5 m (SR) – measuring running speed agility. A detailed description of the Eurofit Test Battery is given in the Council of Europe Handbook for the Eurofit Tests of Physical Fitness [20].

(2) *Gymnastic-specific performance tests.* Gymnastic-specific strength and flexibility tests were developed based on the primary muscle actions principally used in gymnastics as outlined by Carrasco [21]. These actions are: shoulder flexion and shoulder extension, and flexion and extension of the hips. Four strength measures were developed: isometric strength of the shoulders in flexion (SSF); isometric strength of the shoulders in extension (SSE); isometric strength of the hip flexion (SHF); and isometric strength of the hip extension

Table 4. ANOVA results between the different body composition formulae in female gymnasts (n = 84)

Variable	F value	Mean contrasts[a]					
% Fat	208.38**	11.1 (No. 6)	14.6 (No. 4)	15.7 (No. 3)	16.9 (No. 5)	18.8 (No. 1)	19.2 (No. 2)
Fat mass, kg	137.90**	3.7 (No. 6)	5.0 (No. 4)	5.3 (No. 3)	5.5 (No. 5)	6. 3 (No. 1)	6.6 (No. 2)
Fat-free mass, kg	137.90**	26.2 (No. 2)	26.5 (No. 1)	26.6 (No. 5)	27.4 (No. 3)	27.7 (No. 4)	28.5 (No. 6)

[a] The underlined means do not differ significantly (p < 0.01).
** p < 0.01.

(SHE). All these tests were scored in kilograms. In addition four specific flexibility tests were taken: flexibility of the shoulders flexion (FSF); flexibility of the shoulders extension (FSE); flexibility of the hip flexion (FHF); and flexibility of the hip extension (FHE). Each of the flexibility tests were measured as angles and scored in degrees (°). For a full description of these tests refer to Demey [22].

Statistical Analysis

Descriptive statistics (means and SDs) for all variables were calculated for the whole group of gymnasts under study. In order to compare the different body composition formulae, an ANOVA and Pearson product-moment correlations were used. Relations between the body composition estimates (% fat, fat mass, fat-free mass, sum of 6 skinfolds and resistance), and the motor ability tests and the gymnastic-specific strength and flexibility measures were also analyzed by means of Pearson correlations. For all analyses, the SAS programs were used [23]. A significance at the 1% confidence level was accepted.

Results

Descriptive Statistics

Means and standard deviations for the anthropometric and body composition characteristics obtained by the different prediction equations, are given in table 2. Descriptive statistics for the fitness and the gymnastic-specific strength and flexibility tests are illustrated in table 3.

Comparisons between the Different Prediction Equations

As analyzed by an ANOVA for repeated measurements, a significant F-value could be observed for both % fat, fat mass, and fat-free mass, indicating significant differences between the mean values for each respective body composition component (table 4). Mean contrasts revealed that for % fat, signifi-

Table 5. Correlations between the different body composition formulae for % fat, fat mass, and fat-free mass, and SUM6 and RES in female gymnasts (n = 84)

Formulae	No. 1	No. 2	No. 3	No. 4	No. 5	SUM 6	RES
SUM6 skinfolds						–	–0.14
% Fat							
Guo (No. 1)	–					0.85	–0.03
Deurenberg (No. 2)	0.75	–				0.68	–0.47
Houtkooper (No. 3)	0.80	0.77	–			0.80	–0.17
Houtkooper (No. 4)	0.85	0.85	0.78	–		0.76	–0.16
Slaughter (No. 5)	0.79	0.59	0.74	0.69	–	0.95	–0.04
Thorland (No. 6)	0.85	0.75	0.83	0.78	0.85	0.96	–0.20
Fat mass							
Guo (No. 1)	–					0.74	–0.53
Deurenberg (No. 2)	0.96	–				0.62	–0.64
Houtkooper (No. 3)	0.96	0.95	–			0.75	–0.52
Houtkooper (No. 4)	0.96	0.94	0.94	–		0.76	–0.47
Slaughter (No. 5)	0.94	0.91	0.92	0.90	–	0.80	–0.51
Thorland (No. 6)	0.96	0.94	0.96	0.94	0.96	0.80	–0.53
Fat-free mass							
Guo (No. 1)	–					0.37	–0.79
Deurenberg (No. 2)	0.99	–				0.41	–0.78
Houtkooper (No. 3)	0.99	0.99	–			0.36	–0.79
Houtkooper (No. 4)	0.99	0.99	0.99	–		0.34	–0.79
Slaughter (No. 5)	0.99	0.98	0.99	0.98	–	0.31	–0.78
Thorland (No. 6)	0.85	0.99	0.99	0.99	0.99	0.36	–0.77

$p \leq 0.01 \rightarrow r \geq 0.29$.

cant higher values were obtained with the equation of Guo et al. [14] (No. 1) and of Deurenberg et al. [15] (No. 2), with mean values of 18.8 and 19.2%, respectively, which do not differ from each other. Lowest values were obtained by the equations of Thorland et al. [19] (No. 6) and of Houtkooper et al. [17] (No. 4), with mean values of 11.1 and 14.6%, respectively. A difference of 8.1% of body fat between the lowest and highest mean values can be observed. For fat mass the same rank order within the different equations as seen for % fat can be observed, with a lowest mean value of 3.7 kg as estimated by the equation of Thorland et al. [19] (No. 6), and a highest mean value of 6.6 kg as estimated by the equation of Deurenberg et al. [15] (No. 2). All mean values differ significantly from each other, except for the equations 3

Table 6. Correlations between body composition characteristics and Eurofit tests in female gymnasts (n = 84)

	FB	PT	SR	SBJ	HG	SU	BAH	SR
SUM 6 skinfolds	0.19	−0.05	−0.16	−0.06	0.23	−0.30	−0.30	0.03
Resistance	0.42	0.57	−0.53	−0.69	−0.66	−0.55	−0.28	0.60
% Fat								
Guo (No. 1)	0.14	−0.15	−0.14	0.01	0.24	−0.20	−0.28	−0.00
Deurenberg (No. 2)	−0.26	−0.52	0.31	0.48	0.66	0.26	−0.01	−0.40
Houtkooper (No. 3)	0.06	−0.17	0.02	0.07	0.34	−0.11	−0.22	−0.08
Houtkooper (No. 4)	−0.03	−0.27	0.04	0.19	0.34	0.01	−0.10	−0.11
Slaughter (No. 5)	−0.18	−0.01	−0.19	−0.11	0.16	−0.34	−0.26	−0.02
Thorland (No. 6)	0.14	−0.13	−0.05	0.03	0.33	−0.22	−0.26	−0.04
Fat mass								
Guo (No. 1)	−0.19	−0.56	0.26	0.51	0.76	0.20	−0.02	−0.47
Deurenberg (No. 2)	−0.31	−0.63	0.40	0.63	0.85	0.34	0.07	−0.57
Houtkooper (No. 3)	−0.18	−0.51	0.28	0.47	0.75	0.16	−0.03	−0.44
Houtkooper (No. 4)	−0.19	−0.51	0.25	0.47	0.71	0.19	−0.01	−0.40
Slaughter (No. 5)	−0.15	−0.47	0.20	0.43	0.69	0.11	−0.01	−0.42
Thorland (No. 6)	−0.13	−0.47	0.23	0.44	0.72	0.11	−0.02	−0.42
Fat-free mass								
Guo (No. 1)	−0.44	−0.74	0.53	0.79	0.90	0.53	0.18	−0.73
Deurenberg (No. 2)	−0.42	−0.74	0.50	0.78	0.90	0.50	0.16	−0.72
Houtkooper (No. 3)	−0.44	−0.75	0.52	0.80	0.90	0.54	0.19	−0.73
Houtkooper (No. 4)	−0.43	−0.74	0.52	0.78	0.89	0.52	0.17	−0.73
Slaughter (No. 5)	−0.45	−0.74	0.55	0.80	0.90	0.56	0.23	−0.74
Thorland (No. 6)	−0.44	−0.74	0.53	0.79	0.90	0.53	0.22	−0.73

$p \leq 0.01 \rightarrow r \geq 0.29$.

and 5. As expected, for fat-free mass, the lowest mean value (= 26.2 kg) was observed for the equation of Deurenberg et al. [15] (No. 2) and a highest mean value (= 28.5 kg) was estimated by the equation of Thorland et al. [19] (No. 6). Except for equations 3 and 5, which do not differ significantly, all fat-free mass mean values differ significantly from each other.

Correlation coefficients between the different body composition equations for % fat, fat mass and fat-free mass are given in table 5. High correlations ($r > 0.90$) can be observed for fat mass and fat-free mass, except for fat-free mass between the equations of Guo et al. [14] and Thorland et al. [19] ($r = 0.85$). Somewhat lower correlations are seen for % fat, with r varying from 0.59 to 0.85.

Table 7. Correlations between body composition characteristics and gymnastic-specific tests in female gymnasts (n = 84)

	SSF	SSE	SHF	SHE	FSF	FSE	FHF	FHE
SUM 6 skinfolds	0.15	0.10	0.11	0.21	0.04	0.29	0.07	0.04
Resistance	-0.76	-0.76	-0.78	-0.75	-0.17	-0.06	-0.32	-0.27
% Fat								
Guo (No. 1)	0.15	0.08	0.09	0.16	0.25	0.15	0.01	0.01
Deurenberg (No. 2)	0.61	0.57	0.59	0.60	0.19	0.29	0.17	0.10
Houtkooper (No. 3)	0.21	0.14	0.20	0.26	0.24	0.11	0.01	0.03
Houtkooper (No. 4)	0.31	0.25	0.27	0.29	0.20	0.25	0.02	0.04
Slaughter (No. 5)	0.10	0.04	0.04	0.15	0.27	0.03	0.10	0.02
Thorland (No. 6)	0.22	0.18	0.20	0.28	0.28	0.09	0.09	0.05
Fat mass								
Guo (No. 1)	0.66	0.61	0.61	0.66	0.19	0.24	0.21	0.16
Deurenberg (No. 2)	0.77	0.74	0.75	0.76	0.15	0.26	0.25	0.17
Houtkooper (No. 3)	0.61	0.57	0.59	0.64	0.20	0.21	0.17	0.15
Houtkooper (No. 4)	0.63	0.58	0.58	0.61	0.19	0.26	0.13	0.14
Slaughter (No. 5)	0.61	0.57	0.56	0.63	0.23	0.17	0.27	0.17
Thorland (No. 6)	0.60	0.57	0.57	0.63	0.24	0.19	0.22	0.16
Fat-free mass								
Guo (No. 1)	0.87	0.85	0.86	0.85	0.04	0.25	0.29	0.22
Deurenberg (No. 2)	0.86	0.84	0.84	0.84	0.05	0.25	0.29	0.22
Houtkooper (No. 3)	0.88	0.86	0.86	0.86	0.04	0.26	0.31	0.22
Houtkooper (No. 4)	0.86	0.84	0.85	0.85	0.04	0.24	0.32	0.22
Slaughter (No. 5)	0.87	0.86	0.86	0.85	0.08	0.29	0.27	0.24
Thorland (No. 6)	0.87	0.86	0.86	0.85	0.09	0.28	0.29	0.24

$p \leq 0.01 \rightarrow r \geq 0.29$.

Relation between Body Composition and Physical Fitness Tests

Correlation coefficients between physical fitness tests, as measured by the Eurofit Test Battery, and body composition variables, as obtained by different prediction equations, are given in table 6. For % fat and fat mass, different correlation values with the respective fitness variables could be observed for the different prediction equations. For the fat-free mass, however, comparable correlation values were obtained for the different equations with each of the different fitness test respectively. A number of fitness variables, especially handgrip (HG) is significantly and positively correlated with % fat estimated by the equations of Deurenberg et al. [15] (No. 2), Houtkooper et al. [16] (No. 3 and 4), and Thorland et al. [19] (No. 6). Other fitness items, such as

Plate tapping (PT), Sit and Reach (SR), Standing Broad Jump (SBJ), and Shuttle Run (SR) are only significantly correlated with % fat as estimated by the Deurenberg et al. [15] equation (No. 2). Moderate to relatively high correlations were observed between fat mass, as estimated by the different equations, and Plate Tapping (r varies from –0.47 to –0.63), Standing Broad Jump (r varies from 0.43 to 0.63), Handgrip (r varies from 0.69 to 0.85), and Shuttle Run (r varies from –0.42 to –0.57). When the Deurenberg et al. [15] equation (No. 2) was used, also significant, moderate correlation values could be observed between fat mass and Flamingo balance (r = –0.31), Sit and Reach (r = 0.40), and Sit-ups (r = 0.34). Moderate to high correlations were observed between all fitness variables (except for Bent Arm Hang) and the fat-free mass component, as estimated by all the equations used.

Relation between Body Composition and Gymnastic-Specific Tests

Correlation values between gymnastic-specific strength and flexibility tests, and % fat, fat mass, and fat-free mass, as estimated by different prediction equations, are given in table 7. No significant, and rather low correlations were observed between all flexibility tests and the body composition components. For the strength items, relatively high, positive correlations with % fat, as estimated by the Deurenberg et al. [15] equation, are seen with r varying from 0.57 to 0.61. Strength, and % fat, as estimated by the other equations, are not significantly correlated, except for the Houtkooper et al. [17] formula (No. 4) where rather low values could be observed with SSF (0.31) and SHE (0.29). Significant and relatively high, positive correlations are observed between the four strength measures and the fat mass (r varying from 0.57 to 0.77), and the fat-free mass (r varying from 0.84 to 0.87) components, as estimated by the six equations used.

Discussion

Compared to their age-related peer group of Flemish reference girls [24], the gymnasts are rather small, light, and have less subcutaneous fat development. This is demonstrated by profiling their mean values of stature, weight, and skinfolds relative to the reference percentile norms, with p values of P20 and P26 for stature and weight, respectively, and percentiles varying from P20 to P33 for the skinfold values (table 8). If this sample is compared with world class female gymnasts (mean age: 16.5 + 1.8 years), measured at the 24th World Championships in Artistic Gymnastics, Rotterdam, The Netherlands [8], their mean stature and weight can be profiled around the P3 value. Their mean skinfold values are situated around the P75–P85 values, except for the subscap-

Table 8. Profiling (percentiles) of the gymnasts' sample relative to age-related peers (REF) and elite female gymnasts (GYM) for anthropometric variables and physical fitness tests

Variable	REF [24]	GYM [8]
Anthropometry		
Body weight	P26	P3
Stature	P20	P3
Triceps skinfold	P26	P80
Biceps skinfold	P20	P75
Subscapular skinfold	P25	P25
Suprailiac skinfold	P33	P75
Calf skinfold	P20	P85
Eurofit Test Battery		
Flamingo Balance	P80	–
Plate Tapping	P60	–
Sit and Reach	P95	–
Standing Broad Jum	P88	–
Handgrip	P70	–
Sit-ups	P98	–
Bent Arm Hang	P98	–
Shuttle Run	P91	–

ular mean, which is around the P25 value (table 8). Therefore, subjects in this study have, on average, a morphological build which is characteristic of 'sub-elite' female gymnasts, as seen in the literature [7]. Despite their rather small body size, subjects in this study performed very well on fitness tests, comprising the Eurofit Test Battery. Compared to their age-related peers for the different fitness variables, mean values are situated around the P60 and even P98 values, for Plate Tapping, and Sit-ups and Bent Arm Hang, respectively (table 8).

The use of different prediction equations using both BIA estimates or skinfolds as independant variables, results in significantly different body composition estimates in this sample (table 4). For % fat and fat mass, highest mean values were obtained by the equation of Deurenberg et al. [15] (No. 2) and lowest values by the equation of Thorland et al. [19] (No. 6), with means of 19.2% and 6.6 kg, and 11.1% and 3.7 kg, respectively, resulting in mean differences of 8.1% in percentage of body fat and 2.9 kg in fat mass. For fat-free mass, opposite results were obtained. A lowest mean value was obtained by the equation of Deurenberg et al. [15] (mean = 26.2 kg) and the highest mean value was obtained when the equation of Thorland et al. [19] was used (mean = 28.5 kg). This resulted in a significant mean difference of 2.3 kg of fat-free mass. Although significantly different mean values were obtained, high correlations were observed between the different equations for the fat mass and fat-free mass components (r varying from 0.85 to 0.99). The correlations for % fat are somewhat lower (r varying from 0.59 to 0.85), especially between the Slaughter et al. [18] equation (No. 5) and the equations of Deurenberg et al. [15] (No. 2) and Houtkooper et al. [17] (No. 4), with correlation values of r = 0.59 and r = 0.69, respectively (table 5).

The use of different equations resulting in significantly different body composition estimates in this group of gymnasts, is in accordance with the findings of Boileau [25] and of Roemmich et al. [26] in reference children, as well as in female gymnasts in the studies of Claessens et al. [27], Eckerson et al. [28], and Housh et al. [29]. Comparing five skinfold equations in a group of 153 female gymnasts (mean age = 16.4 ± 1.7 years), who participated at the 24th World Championship Artistic Gymnastics held in Rotterdam The Netherlands in 1987, Claessens et al. [27] found a mean difference of 7% of body fat percentage between the highest (14.1% fat) and lowest (7.1% fat) mean values. A mean difference of 6% of body fat could also be observed in a group of 73 Caucasian high school female gymnasts (mean age = 15.7 ± 1.2 years) between the highest (22.9% fat) and lowest (16.9% fat) mean values in comparing eleven skinfold equations [29]. If BIA equations were compared in the same group of high school female gymnasts, a mean difference of 9.4 kg in fat-free mass between the highest (44.2 kg) and lowest (34.8 kg) mean values was demonstrated [28].

Each of the equations used were validated and/or cross-validated against a 'criterion' body composition method (commonly the hydrostatic weighing technique), and thus, from a 'methodological' point of view, were valuable [28, 29]. However, from a 'practical' point of view, the question arises as to which of these prediction equations can best be used in the practical setting of the gymnastic environment?

To answer this question, a number of 'external' criteria were used against which the six formulae were compared and 'evaluated', that is (1) the sum of six skinfolds (SUM6) was used as a total amount of body fatness; (2) how do the body composition parameters as estimated by the different equations correlate with the fitness and performance tests?; (3) what is the best equation from a practical point of view, based on the criteria of applicability?; and (4) are there some 'health' consequences associated with the use of certain equations?

Using the sum of six skinfolds (SUM6) as a total body fat criterion can be justified by the fact that the development of subcutaneous fatness, or 'visible fatness', is more important than total fatness in esthetic sports, such as gymnastics. It is also recognized that in children the 'sum of skinfolds' is preferable as an indicator of fatness compared to regression equations. This is because of the invalid 'transformations' that are made based on the assumed 'constancy' of the fat-free mass component in children [25, 26, 30–32]. Correlations between the different body composition equations and SUM6 range from $r=0.68$ to $r=0.96$ for % fat; from $r=0.62$ to $r=0.80$ for fat mass; and from $r=0.31$ to $r=0.41$ for fat-free mass. It can be argued that equations from which % fat and fat mass correlations are 'high', and fat-free mass correlates 'low' with SUM6, give the 'best' results. Based on this principle, it may be suggested that both 'skinfold' equations (No. 5 and 6) give the 'best' results, followed by the 'BIA' formulae, from which the formula of Deurenberg et al. [15] (No. 2) provide the 'worst' results. This is also confirmed by the correlations between % fat and the resistance parameter, where a relatively high negative correlation is found when the Deurenberg et al. [15] formula is used ($r=-0.47$). With the other equations, correlation values ranging from $r=-0.03$ to $r=-0.20$ were obtained (table 5).

Another 'external' criterion is to look to the relationship between the body composition estimates obtained by the different equations, and the fitness and performance tests. In sports, the fat-free mass component is an important body composition characteristic. It can be argued that a certain body composition equation which reveals higher correlations between its derived fat-free mass component and several motor ability and gymnastic-specific strength and flexibility measures, can be considered as the 'best' prediction equation. Based on the correlations between the fat-free mass, as estimated by the six equations, and the Eurofit tests (table 6) and the gymnastic-specific tests (table 7), it can be stated that none of the six equations provided appropriate results. For all equations, comparable correlation values were obtained with each of the motor and performance tests, respectively. If SUM6 is taken as the 'criterion', it can be argued that 'comparable' correlations values between % fat and fat mass, as obtained with the six equations, and the fitness and performance measures, respectively, has to be obtained. Based on this argument, it is clearly demonstrated that the correlations provided by the Houtkooper et al. [16] equation (No. 4), and especially the Deurenberg et al. [15] equation (No. 2) do not 'correspond' with the correlation values received by the other equations. From this point of view, both prediction equations provide poor results compared to the others.

One of the primary purposes in developing regression equations is to assess an individuals' body composition in the field. As a consequence, the 'best' equation is characterized by a relatively small number of independent variables which can be taken easily on the subject. From a subject's perspective, the chosen measurements have to fulfil the criteria of applicability [33, 34]. Although bioelectrical impedance measurements principally meet the needs of this criterion, it is also demonstrated that in practice, BIA body composition estimates in general, and especially in children, are not as accurate and reliable as believed [13, 35]. Characteristics such as posture, the length of time a subject is recumbent, the abduction of limbs, consumption of food or beverages, recent exercise, and the hydration status, including hydration to the menstrual cycle in females, affects the BIA measures [35]. Therefore, the BIA method may be less applicable compared to skinfolds. The measurement of most skinfolds is relatively straightforward for both the tester and subject. Therefore, it may be argued that the use of 'skinfold' equations is preferable to 'BIA' equations.

Another criterion related to choice of equation is its 'health' consequences. To reach a high level in artistic gymnastics, a 'gymnastic'-specific morphological make-up is preferred. A very low level of fatness, both total and subcutaneous, is a primary concern [7]. Female gymnasts are often pushed by their parents and/or coaches to maintain, or reduce their body weight, in order to attain an 'ideal' body form [36]. This can lead to physical and psychological health problems. From this point of view, prediction equations which produce high(er) % fat estimates, as compared to those which give comparable results within the gymnastic population, are not the best choice. Based on this argument, the equations of Deurenberg et al. [15] (No. 2) and Guo et al. [14] (No. 1), which produced significantly higher mean values for % fat and fat mass, compared to the other four equations, are not preferred.

In conclusion, the choice of the best equation to predict body composition characteristics in young female gymnasts is not a simple task. An initial prerequisite is that the equation should be valid and must meet the needs of specificity and cross-validity [37]. Although such gymnastic-specific equations are available for young female gymnasts [28, 29], from a practical point of view, not all are appropriate. Based on the 'external' criteria used in this study, it can be concluded that the 'skinfold' equations are to be preferred. The 'choice' between skinfold equations depends of the preference of the tester. If subjects acceptability is the most important factor, the Slaughter et al. [18] equation (No. 5) is best, because only two skinfolds (triceps and calf) need to be taken. If 'low' % fat values are preferable, the Thorland et al. [19] equation (No. 6) is the best choice. However, considering all of the 'problems' associated with the 'development' and 'applicability' of regression equations to predict body composition characteristics, especially during the growing period, a sum of skinfolds in conjunction with the height and weight is recommended, rather than reporting an errant % fat [26]. As an additional reference, extended gymnastic-specific anthropometric profile charts for female (and male) gymnasts are available [8].

References

1   Malina RM: Growth and Maturation of Female Gymnasts. Spotlight on Youth Sports. East Lansing, Institute for the Study of Youth Sports, Michigan State University, 1996 vol 19, pp 1–3.
2   Bar-Or O (ed): The Child and Adolescent Athlete. Oxford, Blackwell Scientific, 1996.
3   Carter JEL, Heath BH: Somatotyping: Development and Applications. Cambridge, Cambridge University Press, 1990.
4   Claessens AL: Talent detection and talent development: Kinanthropometric issues. Acta Kinesiol Univ Tartuensis 1999;4:47–64.
5   Malina RM: Talent Identification and Selection in Sport. Spotlight on Youth Sports. East Lansing, Institute for the Study of Youth Sports, Michigan State University, 1997, vol 20, pp 1–3.
6   Normile D: Where is women's gymnastics going? Int Gymnast 1996;38:46–47.
7   Claessens AL: Elite female gymnasts: A kinanthropometric overview; in Johnston FE, Eveleth P, Zemel B (eds): Human Growth in Context. London, Smith-Gordon, 1999, pp 273–280.
8   Claessens AL, Veer FM, Stijnen V, Lefevre J, Maes H, Steens G, Beunen G: Anthropometric characteristics of outstanding male and female gymnasts. J Sports Sci 1991;9:53–74.
9   American College of Sports Medicine: The Female Athlete Triad. Position Stand. Med Sci Sports Exerc 1997;29:i–ix.
10 O'Connor PJ, Lewis RD, Boyd A: Health concerns of artistic women gymnasts. Sports Med 1996; 21:321–325.
11 Roche AF, Heymsfield SB, Lohman TG (eds): Human Body Composition. Champaign, Human Kinetics, 1996.
12 Claessens AL, Beunen G, Malina RM: Anthropometry, physique, body composition, and maturity assessment; in Armstrong N, Van Mechelen W (eds): Textbook of Paediatric Exercise Science and Medicine. Oxford, Oxford University Press, 2000, in press.
13 National Institute of Health Technology: Bioelectrical impedance analysis in body composition measurement: Assessment Conference Statement. Am J Clin Nutr 1996;64(suppl):524S-532S.
14 Gou S, Roche AF, Chumlea WC, Miles DS, Pohlman RL: Body composition predictions from bioelectrical impedance. Hum Biol 1987;59:221–234.
15 Deurenberg P, Kusters CSL, Smit HE: Assessment of body composition in children and young adults is strongly age-dependent. Eur J Clin Nutr 1990;44:261–268.
16 Houtkooper LB, Going SB, Lohman TG, Roche AF, Van Loan M: Bioelectrical impedance estimation of fat-free body mass in children and youth: A cross-validation study. J Appl Physiol 1992;72:366–373.
17 Houtkooper LB, Lohman TG, Going SB, Hall MC: Validity of bioelectrical impedance for body composition assessment in children. J Appl Physiol 1989;66:814–821.
18 Slaughter MH, Lohman TG, Boileau RA, Horswill CA, Stillman RJ, Van Loan MD, Bemben DA: Skinfold equations for estimation of body fatness in children and youth. Hum Biol 1988;60:709–723.
19 Thorland WG, Johnson GO, Tharp GD, Housh TJ, Cisar CJ: Estimation of body density in adolescent athletes. Hum Biol 1984;56:439–445.
20 Council of Europe: European Test of Physical Fitness. Handbook for the Eurofit Tests of Physical Fitness. Rome, Council of Europe, Committee for the Development of Sport, 1988.
21 Carrasco R: Gymnastique aux Agrès. L'Activité du Débutant. Paris, Vigot Frères, 1975.
22 Demey S: Strength and flexibility characteristics in female gymnasts (in Dutch); Master Thesis, Faculty of Physical Education and Physiotherapy, Katholieke Universiteit Leuven, Belgium, 1993.
23 SAS Institute Inc: Statistical Analysis System Procedures Guide, Release 6.03 Edition. Cary, SAS Institute, 1988.
24 Lefevre J, Beunen G, Borms J, Vrijens J, Claessens AL, Van der Aerschot H: Eurofit Testbattery. Reference values for 6–12 year, and growth curves for 6–18 year old boys and girls in Flanders (in Dutch). Gent, Publicatiefonds voor Lichamelijke Opvoeding, 1993.
25 Boileau RA: Body composition assessment in children and youths; in Bar-Or O (ed): The Child and Adolescent Athlete. Oxford, Blackwell Publications, 1996, pp 523–537.
26 Roemmich JN, Clark PA, Weltman A, Rogol AD: Alterations in growth and body composition during puberty. I. Comparing multicompartment body composition models. J Appl Physiol 1997; 83:927–935.

27 Claessens AL, Lefevre J, Beunen G, Maes H, Stijnen V, Veer AMJ, Garcet L: A comparison of different prediction equations in determining body composition of outstanding female gymnasts; in Ellis KJ, Eastman JD (eds): Human Body Composition. New York, Plenum Press, 1993, pp 83–84.

28 Eckerson JM, Evetovich TK, Stout JR, Housh TJ, Johnson GO, Housh DJ, Ebersole KT, Smith DB: Validity of bioelectrical impedance equations for estimating fat-free mass weight in high school female gymnasts. Med Sci Sports Exerc 1997;29:962–968.

29 Housh TJ, Johnson GO, Housh DJ, Eckerson JM, Stout JR: Validity of skinfold estimates of percent fat in high school female gymnasts. Med Sci Sports Exerc 1996;28:1331–1335.

30 Wang ZM, Deurenberg P, Wang W, Pietrobelli A, Baumgartner RN, Heymsfield SB: Hydration of fat-free body mass: A review and critique of a classic body composition constant. Am J Clin Nutr 1999;69:833–841.

31 Wells JCK, Fuller NJ, Dewit O, Fewtrell MS, Elia M, Cole TJ: Four-component model of body composition in children: Density and hydration of fat-free mass and comparison with simpler models. Am J Clin Nutr 1999;69:904–914.

32 Withers RT, Laforgia J, Heymsfield SB: Critical appraisal of the estimation of body composition via two-, three-, and four-compartment models. Am J Hum Biol 1999;11:175–185.

33 Cameron N: The Measurement of Human Growth. London, Croom Helm, 1984.

34 Micozzi MS: Applications of anthropometry to epidemiologic studies of nutrition and cancer. Am J Hum Biol 1990;2:727–739.

35 Kushner RF, Gudivaka R, Schoeller DA: Clinical characteristics influencing bioelectrical impedance analysis measurements. Am J Clin Nutr 1996;64(suppl):423S–427S.

36 Rosen LW, Hough DO: Pathogenic weight-control behaviors of female college gymnasts. Phys Sports Med 1988;16:141–144.

37 Katch FI, Katch VL: Measurement and prediction errors in body composition assessment and the search for the perfect prediction equation. Res Q Exerc Sport 1980;51:249–260.

Prof. Dr. A.L. Claessens, Katholieke Universiteit Leuven,
Faculty of Physical Education and Physiotherapy, Department of Sports and Movement Sciences,
Tervuursevest, 101, B-3001 Heverlee (Leuven) (Belgium)
Tel. +32 016 32.90.83, Fax +32 016 32.91.97, E-Mail albrecht.claessens@flok.kuleuven.ac.be

Jürimäe T, Hills AP (eds): Body Composition Assessment in Children and Adolescents.
Med Sport Sci. Basel, Karger, 2001, vol 44, pp 155–167

··························

Longitudinal Relationship between the Development of Body Fat Mass in Adolescent Males and Females and Their Eating and Activity Pattern

H.C.G. Kemper, W. van Mechelen, G.B. Post, J.W.R. Twisk, W. de Vente

AGAHLS Research Group, EMGO Institute, Amsterdam, The Netherlands

Since the 1960s there has been an increase in the prevalence of obesity not only in adults but also in youth. This increase has occurred in North America [1] and Europe. In the Netherlands the prevalence of obesity (BMI > 30) in 1997 was estimated as 7% for adult men and as 11% for adult women [2]. The increase is also discernable in youth [3]. In US adolescents aged 12–17 years, the increase in the prevalence of obesity measured with triceps skinfold between 1963 and 1980 was about 18% in boys and 21% in girls. Additionally, there seems to be a clear relation between obesity and other biological risk indicators of cardiovascular diseases (CVD) [4] such as hypertension, hypercholesterolemia and noninsulin-dependent diabetes mellitus (NIDDM). Obesity during childhood and adolescence is reported to be an important determinant of adult obesity [5]. Guo et al. [6] found that 40% of children who were obese at age 7 years of age became obese adults, and more than 70% of obese adolescents remained obese as adults.

Apart from biological indicators [7], many lifestyle factors are associated with the development of obesity in youth. Important lifestyles in this respect are physical activity, dietary intake, smoking, drinking and early events in fetal and infantile growth. Most prevention programs are focussed on healthy diets and a more physically active life because these two lifestyles are thought to be of major importance in the development of obesity. Therefore, the successful prevention of obesity must be started as early as possible in the growing years and focus on dietary habits and habitual physical activity.

In this paper, the results of a longitudinal study are presented. A group of healthy 13-year-old adolescents were followed over a period of 15 years till age 27 years and relationships between the group's daily dietary intake and daily physical activity and the development of body fat (as a risk indicator for CVD) were explored. The major goals of this study were to determine: (1) the longitudinal influence of two lifestyle factors on the development of obesity, and (2) the amount of tracking of physical activity, dietary patterns and obesity over time in young males and females. The data in this paper were collected as part of the Amsterdam Growth and Health Longitudinal Study (AGAHLS) [8, 9].

Methods

The Amsterdam Growth and Health Longitudinal Study (AGAHLS) used a multiple longitudinal design in which repeated measurements were made in three birth cohorts (1962, 1963 and 1964) of males and females [8, 9]. The subjects were recruited as a whole sample from a secondary school in Amsterdam. Between 1976 and 1998, eight repeat measurements were completed: during the school period (13–17 years) four annual measurements, a fifth in 1985 (mean age 21 years), a sixth and seventh measurement in 1991 and 1993 (mean ages 27 and 29 years) and an eighth measurement in 1996/1997 (mean age 33 years). Over the 15–year period the total drop-out rate was 40%.

Anthropometric measurements of body height, body mass and four skinfolds (biceps, triceps, subscapular and suprailiac) were performed according standard procedures [10]. Fat mass was estimated as a percentage of body fat from the sum of four skinfolds (mm) and body mass (kg) according to Durnin and Rahaman [11]. Body mass index (BMI), being the ratio between body mass (kg) and body height squared (m^2) is also included as an indirect measure of fat mass, because it is often used in epidemiological research as the only measure of obesity.

In addition to this biological risk indicator for CVD, two lifestyle factors were monitored. Dietary intake (DI) was measured by a modification of the cross-check dietary history interview in a time-frame of the last 3 months [12]. All subjects were interviewed by a dietitian to recall their usual food intake (food and drink) by reporting the frequency (limited to at least twice a month), amounts (with models used to illustrate common portion sizes such as glasses, bowls, spoons and imitations of sizes of potatoes and fruits; a pair of scales to weigh sugar and butter additions) and methods of preparation of the foods consumed during the previous month. During adolescence (13–17 years) the details of several food items (for example, skimmed or whole milk) and preparation (addition of butter and sauce to vegetables and meat) are questioned with the parents. All consumed food items were transformed into nutrients by the Dutch Food and Nutrition Table [13]. The following food characteristics were used: total daily energy intake (relative to body mass) and percentage of energy from carbohydrates, fat and protein.

Physical activity (PA) was measured by a standardized activity interview based on a questionnaire [14]. The interview was retrospective over the previous 3 months and covered the following areas: organized sports activities, unorganized sports activities (for example, playing in the street), active transportation (such as bicycling), and activities at home, school and work.

Only those physical activities maintained for a minimum duration of 5 min and an intensity level of four times basal metabolic rate (4 METs) were considered. The physical activities were classified in three intensity levels, 5.5, 8.5 and 11.5 METs, respectively [15]. The PA score was calculated as the average weekly time (minutes) spent multiplied by the respective level of METs. This weighted energy expenditure was used as the physical activity score of each subject for each year of measurement. Both body composition and lifestyle factors were obtained for each year of data collection by identical procedures in all subjects.

Tracking of both biological and lifestyle risk factors was assessed by stability coefficients from a regression model in which the initial value of a certain indicator is regressed to the entire longitudinal development of that factor. The relationships between the initial value and all other values are tested simultaneously, leading to one standardized regression coefficient (beta), which can be interpreted as a longitudinal correlation coefficient or stability coefficient [16]. In the current analysis, six data points were used (at mean age 13, 14, 15, 16, 21 and 27, respectively). The major advantage of this method is that the stability coefficients are calculated using all available longitudinal data. The magnitude of this stability coefficient ranges from 0 to 1, which makes the coefficient interpretable as a longitudinal correlation coefficient. The magnitude of the stability coefficients was estimated with Generalized Estimating Equations (GEE).

To analyze the effect of lifestyle factors on the longitudinal development of a high fat mass, at each longitudinal measurement point the subjects were divided into two groups with respect to their fat mass. The threshold values were based on the values for percentage of body fat ($>20\%$ for males and $>30\%$ for females) and BMI ($>25 \text{ kg} \cdot \text{m}^{-2}$). The magnitude of the relationship with lifestyle parameters was calculated with a statistical model described previously [17]. The longitudinal relationship between lifestyle factors and high fat mass factors were also analyzed with GEE. With this method, the longitudinal relationships are analyzed by using all available data and under correction of both time-dependent (for example age) and time-independent (for example sex) covariates. The method also takes into account that the repeated observations of each individual are not independent. As a result of these analyses, odds ratios (OR) were calculated which indicated the relationships of obesity with DI and PA over the 15-year period.

In all analyses, a probability level of $p < 0.05$ was accepted as significant. Odds ratio and regression coefficients (beta) are given with a 95% confidence interval (95% CI).

Results

Population Characteristics

In table 1, mean and standard deviations are provided for the main characteristics (anthropometry, measures of fat mass and two lifestyle factors: dietary intake and physical activity) of the males (n = 83) and females (n = 98) at the mean age of 27 years.

The differences between sexes are statistically significant for all anthropometric measures ($p < 0.01$) except for BMI ($p < 0.06$). DI for males showed a

Table 1. Mean and standard deviations of the physical characteristics at the repeated measurement at the mean age of 27 years

	Males (n = 83)		Females (n = 98)		p value
	x̄	SD	x̄	SD	
Body height, cm	183.1	6.4	169.9	7.8	<0.01
Body mass, kg	75.4	8.5	63.3	7.8	<0.01
Sum of 4 skinfolds, mm	36.5	13.5	46.3	16.5	<0.01
Percentage body fat, %	22.3	4.3	25.4	4.6	<0.01
Lean body mass, kg	64.5	6.0	47.5	4.9	<0.01
Body mass index, kg · m^{-2}	22.6	2.2	21.9	2.5	NS
Dietary intake					
Total daily energy intake relative to body mass, kJ · kg^{-1}	170.5	44.1	150.4	39.6	<0.01
Protein intake, en%	13.01	2.2	14.3	2.1	<0.01
Carbohydrate intake, en%	45.2	4.4	43.8	5.3	NS
Fat intake, en%	39.1	4.8	39.6	5.5	NS
Physical activity					
Total weekly physical activity (METs)	2,909	2,262	3,179	1,909	NS

Significant differences between sexes (p < 0.05) are listed in the last column.
NS = Not significant.

significantly higher energy intake and lower percentage of protein intake than females. PA levels showed no significant differences between males and females.

Age Changes of Lifestyles

The longitudinal results of DI between age 13 and 27 years (fig. 1) show a decrease in energy intake per kilogram body mass from about 225 kJ per day at age 13 years to about 155 kJ per day at age 27 years. Boys show a higher energy intake over the adolescent (13–16 years) and young adult period (17–27 years), but in the adolescent period the energy intake is 15% higher than girls and in the young adult period about 10%.

The longitudinal results of PA (fig. 2) show a steep decrease in the energy expenditure in both sexes from age 13 on declining from about 5,000 METs per week to about 3,000 METs per week at age 27 years. During adolescence, boys show a 20% higher energy expenditure than girls but at age 27 there is no significant difference between males and females.

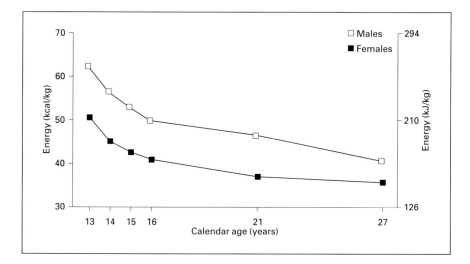

Fig. 1. The longitudinal development of daily dietary intake (mean and standard deviation) in males (n = 89) and females (n = 97) measured as the total energy intake in MJ (kcal) per day between the mean age of 13 and 27 years.

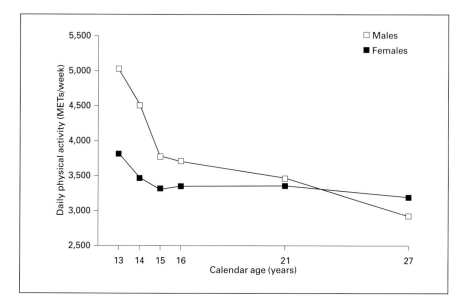

Fig. 2. The longitudinal development of daily physical activity (mean and standard deviation) in males (n = 89) and females (n = 97) measured as the weighted activity score in METs per week between the mean age of 13 and 27 years.

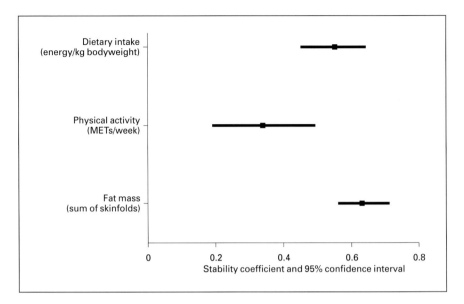

Fig. 3. Stability coefficients (and 95% CI) of dietary intake (energy intake relative to body mass per day), physical activity (METs per week) and fat mass (sum of four skinfolds) in youth over a period of 15 years between age 13 and 27 years.

Tracking Results

Results of tracking analyses over the 15-year period (fig. 3) indicate a low but significant stability coefficient of the lifestyle indicator PA (METs per week) of 0.34 (0.19–0.49), and a higher stability coefficient of DI (energy intake relative to body mass) of 0.55 (0.45–0.64). The stability coefficient of the sum of four skinfolds as a measure of fat mass shows a considerably higher value of 0.63 (0.56–0.71).

Relationship between Lifestyles and Obesity

Which lifestyle factors discriminate between high- and low-risk participants on the basis of fatness? The relationships between DI and a high fat mass (measured as the sum of four skinfolds) resulted in a significant OR of 1.5 (1.2–1.8) with energy intake of protein, but not with the energy intake of fat and carbohydrate. The OR with total energy intake was 0.37 (0.28–0.49), indicating that a relatively high fat mass was significantly related with a low energy intake. With PA (measured as the weighted energetic score) a high fat mass resulted in an OR of 0.81 (0.69–0.96), indicating that a high PA was related to a low fat mass.

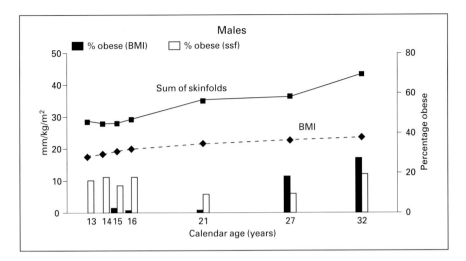

Fig. 4. Longitudinal development of fat mass in males, estimated from sum of 4 skinfolds and BMI between 13 and 32 years. The columns indicate the prevalence of obesity at each year of measurements (>20% body fat; >25 BMI).

Discussion

Prevalence of Obesity

In the study population, the PA, measured as the mean EE, decreases rapidly and the DI measured as the mean EI increases in absolute terms but not relative to fatness during adolescence and young adulthood. The indirect measure of fat mass (sum of 4 skinfolds) increases gradually in both males and females between 13 and 27 years. This change results in an increased prevalence rate of obesity. In males (fig. 4) between 13 and 16 years less than 10% are obese (defined as >20% body fat). At 32 years of age (although not represented in the results) this percentage had doubled to 20%. In females (fig. 5) the percentage increase was greater from about 10% (obese >30% body fat) between 13 and 16 years up to 30% at age 32.

Representativeness of the Study Population

The mean BMI values, measured in 1996/1997, at age 32 were 24.0 (2.6) in males and 22.9 (4.4) in females. These BMI values are almost comparable with recent data from the MORGEN study [18] in which in a random sample of the Dutch population, the prevalence of risk indicators was monitored. In 30- to 34-year-old males and females a mean BMI of 24.3 (3.2) in males and of 23.8 (3.7) in females was reported.

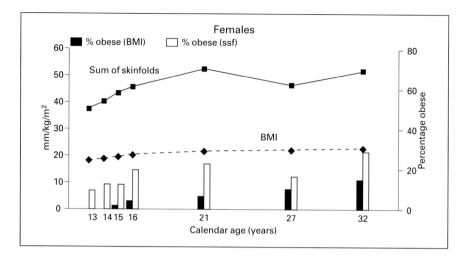

Fig. 5. Longitudinal development of fat mass in females, estimated from sum of 4 skinfolds and BMI between 13 and 32 years. The columns indicate the prevalence of obesity at each year of measurements (>20% body fat; >25 BMI).

The population from the AGAHLS can therefore be considered as representative of the whole Dutch population. Other characteristics such as socio-economic states (SES) showed levels that are only slightly higher than the average Dutch population [8]. Although the prevalence of obesity is about 20–30%, one must take into account that the majority of the males and females do show values for fat mass that are in the normal range and are not overweight or obese according the criteria of the World Health Organization [1]. The trend of an increasing prevalence of obesity in youth is undoubtedly related to the changes in DI and/or PA.

Effects of Repeated Testing

In the AGAHLS, a control group was used by measuring comparable boys and girls from another secondary school in Purmerend. During the four annual measurement periods (1976–1979) all boys and girls from the three birth cohorts (1962, 1963 and 1964) were only measured once. In 1996/1997 this control group was remeasured for a second time after 20 years.

A comparison of the data for fatness and lifestyles of the longitudinal group (8 repeated measurements) and the control group with only 2 repeated measurements (results not reported in the present paper) can give information about this testing effect.

In table 2 the results from this control group and the longitudinal group at age 33/34 years are presented. The percentage of males and females (defined

Table 2. Amsterdam growth and health longitudinal study (1996/1997 results, age 33/34 years)

		Total	Longitudinal	Control
		$(N_{\male}=207/N_{\female}=231)$ %	$(N_{\male}=73/N_{\female}=87)$ %	$(N_{\male}=134/N_{\female}=144)$ %
Obesity	$\male$	27.1	27.4	26.9
(BMI > 25)	$\female$	14.8	14.9	14.7
Obesity	$\male$	18.4	19.4	17.9
(fat % > 20/30)	$\female$	25.5	28.7	23.6

Table 3. Comparison of the control group with the longitudinal group at age 33/34 years in energy intake (kcal/kg) and physical activity (METs)

		Total	Longitudinal	Control
		$(N_{\male}=207/N_{\female}=231)$ %	$(N_{\male}=73/N_{\female}=87)$ %	$(N_{\male}=134/N_{\female}=144)$ %
Energy intake, kcal/kg	$\male$	37.4 (9.9)	35.8 (8.0)	38.2 (10.6)
	$\female$	35.0 (8.6)	35.0 (7.4)	34.9 (9.4)
Physical activity, METs	$\male$	2,972 (2,241)	2,785 (1,906)	3,075 (2,406)
	$\female$	3,125 (2,332)	2,884 (1,532)	3,261 (2,677)

as BMI > 25, fat% > 20/30) are not statistically significant between the control and longitudinal group of both sexes.

The same is true for lifestyles factors measured as energy (kcal/kg) intake and physical activity (table 3).

It was expected that longitudinal repeated testing would result in a selective drop out of subjects who were overweight and/or with more or less unhealthy lifestyles (such as too much dietary intake and low levels of physical activity). However, this was not the case. This result supports the generalizability of these longitudinal results to other comparable populations.

Stability of Fat Mass

The fat mass estimated from the sum of four skinfolds showed a relative high stability over the 15-year period. The stability coefficient is 0.63 and higher than other CVD risk indicators such as diastolic blood pressure (0.34), systolic blood pressure (0.43) and equal to serum cholesterol (0.71) [16]. The high stability of fat mass is an important finding because this knowledge makes it possible to aim intervention towards this biological parameter early in adolescence.

The low stability coefficient of the lifestyle indicator PA demonstrates that physical activity is less stable over the growing years: a boy or girl that has a relatively low or high energy expenditure at age 13 does not necessarily have also a low or a high energy expenditure at age 17, 21 or 27. Part of the low stability may be caused by the lack of reliability of the measurement method of these lifestyles by interview. However, the reproducibility of both interview methods as estimated by interperiod correlations showing that the zero interval of the regression line between 0.7 and 0.8 [19] was found to be acceptable.

Lifestyle in Relation to Obesity

There is little data in the literature on the relationship between the lifestyle factors physical activity (PA) and dietary intake (DI) and obesity in this age group [20].

The literature on the relation between PA and obesity among adolescents gives a variety of results with cross sectional studies reporting inverse relations [21–24]. One intervention study [25] showed no relation and a case-control study resulted in an inverse relation [26].

The reviews by Parizkova [27] and Roberts [28] and the meta-analysis of Ballor and Keessey [29] in general conclude that obesity in adolescents only can be altered by increasing PA and decreasing DI at the same time.

The analysis discriminating subjects with a relatively high and low fat mass resulted in only one biological meaningful significant positive relationship to DI namely protein intake. But, a significant negative relationship was identified with total energy intake, that is, a higher energy intake (per kg body mass) resulted in a relative lower fat mass (OR = 0.37). This unexpected result is not influenced if the nominator (body mass, which includes fat mass) is changed to body height or if energy intake is measured in absolute values. The main reason for this finding may be that the population in general was not obese (see earlier) and that a high total energy intake per se does not necessarily lead to an accumulation of body fat. The other factor in the energy balance equation, energy expenditure also has to be taken into account. The PA, measured as METs per week, showed a negative relationship with fat mass indicating that a higher energy expenditure resulted in lower fat mass (OR = 0.81). A second reason may be the well-known phenomenon of underreporting of DI by the interview method, obese adolescents are prone to 'forget' foodstuffs consumed in order to please the interviewer. A third possibility is the fact that repeated measurements, as in this longitudinal study, can introduce a negative testing effect which was actually found in the boys between age 13 and 16 [19].

% Fat Mass or BMI?

The measurement of body fat by indirect estimations from the sum of four skinfolds or by BMI can also be questioned. The longitudinal relation between fat mass and PA (corrected for differences in DI) showed a significant inverse relationship between the age of 13 and 27 years (beta = –0.08; –0.03 to –0.1) if fat mass was measured as the sum of four skinfolds. This was not the case if fat mass was estimated from BMI (beta = –0.03; –0.06 to 0.01). BMI is an even more indirect estimation of body fat than skinfolds but in large epidemiological studies BMI has the advantage of its simplicity of measurement. BMI has shown high correlations with more direct measurements of obesity and or fat mass. However, BMI and other combinations with body height and body mass are based on a too simple three-component model (muscle, bone and fat) as a measure of body fatness; for instance a variation in muscle (in body builders) and bone (patients with osteoporosis) can influence the BMI.

Moreover, the lean body mass (LBM) also did not show a significant relationship with PA. The longitudinal relation between LBM and PA shows a regression coefficient of 0.00 (–0.02 to 0.02). One should not expect that a high physical activity pattern, by weighing intensity and duration of daily physical activities, should increase the relative amount of muscle mass; physical activities of high intensity and long duration cause training effects that are characterized by slender muscles with a relatively high density of capillarization [20] but the muscles do not show changes in muscle volume hypertrophy.

From this longitudinal data of adolescents and young adults it can be concluded that from age 13 to 27 years, body fatness increases in both sexes resulting in a percentage of obesity between 20 and 30%. Body fatness measured as the sum of four skinfolds indicates a fairly good predictability over the development period of 15 years as indicated by a stability coefficient of 0.63. Of the two lifestyles, PA but not DI is related to a low body fat mass (OR: 0.81). If body fat mass is estimated from BMI however, this relationship can not be demonstrated. Recently, Cole and Roede [30] reported on BMI data that Dutch youth (0–20 years) were thinner than French, American or Norwegian youth, measured up to 20 years earlier based on BMI. Their conclusion, suggesting that the differences in BMI can indicate trends in obesity, may be doubted.

From the present results it can be concluded that promotion of habitual physical activity in the adolescent period seems effective in the early prevention of obesity in young adults.

Acknowledgements

The AGAHLS is supported by multiple grants of the Dutch Prevention Fund, Dutch Heart Foundation, Dutch Ministry of Education and Science, Dutch Ministry of Public Health, Well Being and Sport, the Dairy Foundation on Nutrition and Health and NOC/NSF.

We would like to thank all the men and women who served as our subjects since their early teenage years for their cooperation in the repeated measurements of their growth, health and lifestyles over the past 20 years.

This paper is based on an earlier publication in Int J Obes 1999;23(suppl 3):S34–S40.

References

1   Seidell JC, Rissanen AM: Time trends in the worldwide prevalence of obesity; in Bray GA, Bouchard C, James WPT (eds): Handbook of Obesity. New York, Marcel Dekker, 1998, pp 79–91.
2   Volksgezondheid Toekomst Verkenning 1997: De som der delen (in Dutch). Rijksinstituut voor Volksgezondheid en Milieu. Utrecht, Elsevier/Tijdstroom, 1997.
3   Gortmaker SL, Dietz WH, Sobol AM, Wehler CA: Increasing pediatric obesity in the United States. Am J Dis Child 1987;141:535–540.
4   Després J-P, Moorjani S, Lupien PJ, Tremblay A, Nadeau A, Bouchard C: Regional distribution of body fat, plasma lipoproteins, and cardiovascular disease. Arteriosclerosis 1990;10:497–511.
5   Kolata G: Obese children: A growing problem. Science 1986;232:20–21.
6   Guo SS, Roche AF, Chumlea WC, Gardner JD, Siervogel RM: The predictive value of childhood body mass index values for overweight at age 35 y. Am J Clin Nutr 1994;59:810–819.
7   Bray GA, Bouchard C, James WPT: Handbook of Obesity. New York, Marcel Dekkers, 1998.
8   Kemper HCG (ed): Growth Health and Fitness of Teenagers: Longitudinal Research in International Perspective. Basel, Karger, 1985.
9   Kemper HCG (ed): The Amsterdam Growth Study: A Longitudinal Analysis of Health, Fitness, and Lifestyle. HK Sportscience Monograph. Champaign, Human Kinetics, 1995, vol 6.
10   Weiner JS, Lourie JA: Human Biology: A Guide to Field Methods. IBP Handbook No 9. Oxford, Blackwell, 1969, pp 8–29.
11   Durnin JVGA, Rahaman MM: The assessment of the amount of fat in human body measurements of skinfold thickness. Br J Nutr 1967;21:681–689.
12   Post GB: Nutrition in adolescence: A longitudinal study in dietary patterns from teenager to adult; PhD thesis. Agricultural University of Wageningen, De Vrieseborch, Haarlem, SO, 16, 1989.
13   Dutch Food and Nutrition Table (in Dutch): Zeist, Stichting, NEVO, Voorlichtingsburo voor de Voeding, 1985.
14   Verschuur R: Daily physical activity and health: Longitudinal changes during the teenage period; PhD thesis. University of Amsterdam, De Vrieseborch, Haarlem SO 12, 1987.
15   Montoye HJ, Kemper HCG, Saris WHM, Washburn RA: Measuring Physical Activity and Energy Expenditure. Champaign, Human Kinetics, 1996, pp 123–183.
16   Twisk JWR, Kemper HCG, van Mechelen W, Post GB: Which lifestyle parameters discriminate high- from low-risk participants for coronary heart disease risk factors: Longitudinal analysis covering adolescence and young adulthood. J Cardiovasc Risk 1997;4:393–400.
17   Twisk JWR, Kemper HCG, van Mechelen W, Post GB: Tracking of risk factors for coronary heart disease over a 14-period: A comparison between lifestyle and biologic risk factors with data from the Amsterdam Growth and Health Study. Am J Epidemiol 1997;145:888–898.
18   Blokstra A, Seidell JC, Smit AH, Bueno de Mesquita HB, Verschuren WMM: Morgen Project (in Dutch). Bilthoven, RIVM, 1997.
19   Kemper HCG, van Mechelen W, Post GB, Snel J, Twisk WJR, van Lenthe FJ, Welten DC: The Amsterdam Growth and Health Longitudinal Study, the past (1976–1996) and future (1997–19?). Int J Sports Med 1997;18:S141–S150.

20   Wilmore JH, Costill DL: Physiology of Sport and Exercise. Champaign, Human Kinetics, 1994, pp 223–225.

21   Fripp RR, Hodgson JL, Kwiterovich PO, Werner JC, Schuler HG, Whitman V: Aerobic capacity, obesity and artherosclerotic risk factors in male adolescents. Pediatrics 1985;75:813–817.

22   Pena M, Baccallao J, Barta L, Amador M, Johnston FE: Fiber and exercise in the treatment of obese adolescents. J Adolesc Health Care 1989;10:30–34.

23   Bandini LG, Schoeller DA, Dietz WH: Energy expenditure in obese and nonobese adolescents. Pediatr Res 1990;27:198–203.

24   Roberts SB, Young VR, Fuss P, Heyman MB, Fiatarone M, Dallal GE, Evans WJ: What are the dietary energy needs of elderly adults? Int J Obes 1992;16:969–976.

25   Blaak EE, Westerterp KR, Bar-Or O, Wouters LJM, Saris WHM: Total energy expenditure and spontaneous activity in relation to training in obese boys. Am J Clin Nutr 1992;55:777–782.

26   Moussa MAA, Skaik MB, Yaghy OY, Selwanes SB, Bin-Othman SA: Factors associated with obesity in school children. Int J Obes 1994;18:513–515.

27   Parizkova J: Physical training in weight reduction of obese adolescents. Am J Clin Res 1982;34: 63–68.

28   Roberts SB: Abnormalities of energy expenditure and the development of obesity. Obes Res 1995; 3:1555–1565.

29   Ballor DL, Keessey RE: A meta-analysis of the factors affecting exercise-induced changes in body mass, fat mass and fat-free mass in males and females. Int J Obes 1991;15:717–726.

30   Cole TJ, Roede MJ: Centiles of body mass index for Dutch children aged 0–20 years in 1980: A baseline to assess recent trends in obesity. Ann Hum Biol 1999;26:303–308.

Prof. Dr. Han C.G. Kemper, AGAHLS Research Group, EMGO Institute,
Van der Boechorststraat 7, NL–1081 BT Amsterdam (The Netherlands)
Tel. +31 20 4448407/05, Fax +31 20 4448181, E-Mail hcg.kemper.emgo@med.vu.nl

Jürimäe T, Hills AP (eds): Body Composition Assessment in Children and Adolescents.
Med Sport Sci. Basel, Karger, 2001, vol 44, pp 168–174

....

Validation of Foot to Foot Bioelectrical Impedance in 6- to 10-Year-Old Children

R.A. Abbott, P.S.W. Davies

School of Human Movement Studies, Faculty of Health, Queensland University of
Technology, Kelvin Grove, Brisbane, Queensland, Australia

The measurement of body composition in children requires the use of techniques that are non-invasive and practical as well as precise and accurate. Consequently, some techniques such as in vivo neuron activation or dual X-ray absorptiometry (DXA) can be restricted on ethical grounds, whilst others such as hydrodensitometry, for example, are difficult to undertake in the paediatric population especially in disease states.

Bioelectrical impedance, however, is non-invasive, precise and remarkably simple and straightforward for the subject or patient. As such, the technique has attracted much interest in those wishing to evaluate body composition in childhood [1–5].

The underlying principle of the methodology is that the length^2/impedance (H^2/I) of any conducting medium is proportional to the volume of that conducting medium. In the human, stature is used as a proxy for the length of the conducting medium, that is, the volume of water within the body. The most common method of measuring bioelectrical impedance has been to use four surface electrodes, one attached to the wrist, hand, ankle and foot, respectively. The distal electrodes on each limb are used to induce an 800 µA 50 kHz alternating electrical current within the body. The proximal electrodes measure the voltage drop and bioelectrical impedance can then be calculated. This tetrapolar technique has been validated in children in a number of studies [1, 3, 6]. Recently, however, a variation of the approach has been employed and termed foot to foot or leg to leg bioelectrical impedance analysis. This recent derivation is so named because both the current and the voltage drop are measured via four metallic foot plates which are integrated into a conventional electronic weighing scale. The heels of the foot are placed on two of the plates while the toes and front of the feet are placed on the other two plates. The technique has been validated in a number of studies [7–9] but not, to our knowledge, in children. Some validation studies compare body composition parameters, usually percentage body fat, determined by foot to foot impedance with the same variable determined from a 'gold standard' method, usually DXA or hydrodensitometry. It should be remembered, however, that the index H^2/I is proportional to total body water and any validation study should, in our opinion, compare estimates of total body water from bioelectrical impedance with measures of total body water in the same individuals. We have carried out such an analysis in a cohort of healthy children aged between 6 and 10 years.

Methods

A total of 32 children (12 males and 20 females) aged between 6 and 10 years were recruited from a local school or by advertisement in the local community. The experimental procedures were explained both to the child and the parents or guardian, and written informed consent was obtained from the parent or guardian whilst assent was obtained from the child. The study was approved by the Queensland University of Technology Human Research Ethics Committee. Height was measured to the last completed millimetre using standard procedures. Initially, total body water was predicted via a commercially available foot to foot impedance device. Children were requested to refrain from eating and drink minimally for 2 h prior to measurement. The child stood barefoot on the foot to foot impedance apparatus (Tanita Inc., Tokyo, Japan, model TBF 305) which initially records body weight and when this is stable, predicts total body water via the measurement of impedance and the subjects' height (manually entered into the device). The Tanita TBF 305 also provides results for fat free mass and fat mass estimated from the predicted total body water.

Total body water was then measured in each subject using a stable isotope of oxygen, in the form of water ($H_2^{18}O$). Each subject provided a 10-ml baseline urine sample and then drank a 10% solution of $H_2^{18}O$ based on their body weight (1.0 g/kg body weight). The dose consumed was recorded to two decimal places of a gram. Urine samples were then collected after approximately 5 h and subsequently on a daily basis for 10 days. The enrichment of the predose urine sample, the post dose urine samples, local tap water and the dose given were measured using isotope ratio mass spectrometry (PDZ Europa, Crewe, UK). A 0.5 ml aliquot of each sample to be analysed was placed in a 12-ml exetainer, which were then evacuated for 5 min before being filled with 5% carbon dioxide in nitrogen. The samples were then left at room temperature for 24 h. During this period, equilibrium between the oxygen-18 in the sample and the carbon dioxide gas above the sample was achieved. Reference waters were prepared at the same time and in the same way as the unknown samples. The enrichment of the samples was measured in triplicate. Results were expressed relative to standard mean ocean water (SMOW). The oxygen-18 dilution space (No) was calculated as shown below [10]:

$$No = \frac{TA}{a} \times \frac{(Ea - Et)}{(Es - Ep)},$$

where A is the amount of isotope consumed in grams, a is a portion of that dose in grams retained for mass spectrometric analysis, T is the amount of tap water in which the portion

Table 1. Physical characteristics of the 32 children

	Mean	SD	Range
Age, years	8.24	0.86	6.00–10.10
Height, m	1.312	0.073	1.169–1.547
Weight, kg	30.3	6.6	21.7–50.2

Table 2. Comparison of measured and predicted total body water

	Mean	SD
Total body water (measured), litres	15.85	2.68
Total body water (predicted), litres	18.68	3.77
Bias, litres	2.82	1.89

a is diluted prior to analysis and Ea, Et, and Ep are the isotopic enrichments in delta units relative to SMOW of the portion of the dose, the tap water used and the predose sample. Es is the enrichment in delta units of the intercept of the regression line of the log of the enrichment of the post dose samples and the time of collection in decimal days of those post dose samples relative to the time of dosing. Total body water was then calculated as No/1.01 [11].

The approach of Bland and Altman [12] was used to compare the measured total body water with that predicted by foot to foot impedance. This statistical approach is recognised as the most appropriate way to compare the ability of differing methods to measure the same parameter. The Bland-Altman approach allows for the calculation of the bias between the two techniques. The bias is calculated as being the mean of the differences between the predicted and measured values of total body water.

Results

Some of the physical characteristics of the children studied are shown in table 1. The mean and standard deviation of the measured and predicted total body water and the bias between the measurements are shown in table 2. The mean predicted total body water showed a bias to overestimate measured total body water by, on average, 2.8 litres. However, it should not be assumed that this degree of bias is consistent across the range of measurements made in this study. Figure 1 shows the mean of the two estimates of body water (that is, predicted and measured) plotted against the difference between them.

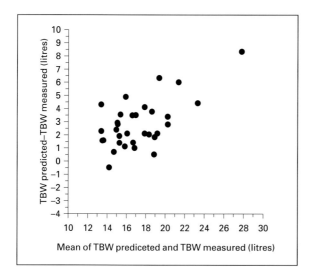

Fig. 1. Bland-Altman plot showing the bias between predicted and measured total body water across the range of measurement.

In the first instance this plot allows the consistency of the bias to be visually assessed. Statistically the correlation between the means and the differences indicates whether there are any trends in the bias. In this case the correlation was highly significant at 0.61 (p<0.05).

Discussion

Foot to foot bioelectrical impedance potentially offers a simple, rapid and acceptable method of assessing body composition in children. Both foot to foot bioelectrical impedance technology and the more longstanding tetrapolar methodology are based on the same fundamental premise that the height^2/impedance of the subject is related to the volume of the conducting medium, that is, total body water. Thus, it is important that validation studies actually measure total body water in order to appropriately assess the ability of any bioelectrical method to predict the same. We have used an oxygen-18 dilution technique to measure in the first instance the oxygen-18 dilution space. This can then be corrected to calculate total body water once an adjustment has been made for the fact that the oxygen-18 dilution space is slightly larger than body water due to the exchange of oxygen with non-aqueous oxygen in the body. The technique is accepted as one of the gold standards for measuring total body water and in vitro tests have shown that in our laboratory the accuracy of oxygen-18 dilution for measuring water volume is approximately 1%.

In comparison with this gold standard, the foot to foot impedance method overestimated body water on average by 2.8 litres or approximately 17% of the measured value. However, it should be noted that as shown in figure 1, the magnitude of the bias is not constant and increases as the measured body water increases. Thus, near the extreme of our current data the foot to foot impedance method is overestimating body water by as much as 6.0 litres or approximately 24% of the true value. In body composition terms this would equate to an error of up to 8 kg in fat-free mass in a child weighing only 37 kg. This would be clearly unacceptable in terms of accuracy.

There are a number of explanations for the apparent difference between total body water as measured using stable isotopes and total body water predicted by foot to foot bioelectrical impedance. Before it is assumed that all the error exists within the impedance methodology the accuracy of the gold standard method used in this study, that is oxygen-18 dilution, should be considered. As stated previously, this technique is widely used to measure body water in both humans and other animals. It is known that oxygen-18 mixes rapidly with total body water and there is some exchange with non-aqueous oxygen. It is assumed in most studies that the overestimation is about 1% and so the oxygen-18 space is reduced by this amount to give total body water. Whilst there will be some physiological variability in the amount of overestimation, that variability is small and is unlikely to produce major error in the final value for total body water.

Technical error can also contribute to total error. Measurements of isotopic enrichment must be both precise and accurate. As we have stated, in vitro experiments have shown that error in the measurement of isotopic enrichment in our laboratory causes an error in the calculation of total body water of less than 1%. Moreover, in this study we have used the so-called back extrapolation method to mathematically calculate body water. As multiple urine samples collected over several days are measured and used in subsequent calculations, this approach is less susceptible to error in comparison with the other mathematical approach, the plateau method, where only one post dose urine sample is collected and measured. Consequently, we have confidence in the isotopic data and the measurement of total body water.

The prediction of total body water from bioelectrical impedance requires that the measured impedance and the conductor length, i.e. measured stature be related to total body water via a regression equation of some description. The exact nature of the equation used within the impedance apparatus is, to the best of our knowledge, unknown. Thus it is difficult to assess the validity of the equation used, however, a bias of 2.5 litres might indicate that the algorithm might be improved. It has been suggested [13] that stature should not be used as a proxy for the conductor length when using foot to foot bioelectrical impedance and that leg length is a more relevant proxy for conductor length. We have been unable to test that particular hypothesis in the current study but it could be argued that as stature and leg length are highly correlated it is unlikely that major improvements in the prediction of total body water would be achieved by using leg length as conductor length. Also it should be noted that we were unable to obtain measurements of bioelectrical impedance and hence total body water in 5 children as the apparatus reported the data as out of range. The common feature of all 5 children is that they all had a low weight for height, i.e. they were thin. This indicates that there are some limitations in the existing software that calculates body composition from measured bioelectrical impedance. Nevertheless, of more concern is the significant correlation seen in figure 1 between the mean of the measurements and their difference. This quite clearly shows that as the volume of body water increases, which we might postulate equates with the child getting physically larger, the error increases dramatically. We have described this phenomenon before [13] with the use of foot to foot impedance in adults and suggested that this finding might be of particular importance when using foot to foot impedance to assess changes in body composition within a weight loss program. In children, the major concern may be the use of the technique in longitudinal studies during which body weight and hence body water would increase as a function of growth.

References

1   Davies PSW, Preece MA, Hicks CJ, Halliday D: The prediction of total body water using bioelectrical impedance in children and adolescents. Ann Hum Biol 1988;15:237–240.
2   Gregory JW, Greene SA, Scrimgeor CM, Rennie MJ: Body water measurement in growth disorders: A comparison of bioelectrical impedance and skinfold thickness with isotope dilution. Arch Dis Child 1991;66:220–222.
3   Danford LC, Schoeller DA, Kushner RF: Comparison of two bioelectrical impedance analysis models for total body water measurements in children. Ann Hum Biol 1992;19:603–607.
4   Ellis KJ, Shypailo RJ, Wong W: Measurement of body water by multifrequency bioelectrical impedance spectroscopy in a multiethnic pediatric population. Am J Clin Nutr 1999;70:847–853.
5   De Lorenzo A, Di Campli C, Andreoli A, Sasso GF, Bonamico M, Gasbarrini A: Assessment of body composition by bioelectrical impedance in adolescent patients with celiac disease. Am J Gastroenterol 1999;94:2951–2955.
6   Mayfield SR, Vavy R, Waldelich D: Body composition of low birthweight infants determined by using bioelectrical resistance and reactance. Am J Clin Nutr 1991;54:296–303.
7   Xie X, Kolthoff N, Barenholt O, Neilsen SP: Validation of leg to leg bioimpedance analysis system in assessing body composition in postmenopausal women. Int J Obes 1999;23:1079–1084.
8   Utter AC, Nieman DC, Ward AN, Butterworth DE: Use of the leg to leg bioelectrical impedance method in assessing body composition change in obese women. Am J Clin Nutr 1999;69:603–607.

9   Nunez C, Gallagher D, Visser M, Pi-Sunyer FX, Wang Z, Heymsfield SB: Bioimpedance analysis: Evaluation of leg to leg system based on pressure constant electrodes. Med Sci Sports Exerc 1996; 29:524–531.

10   Halliday D, Miller AG: Precise measurement of total body water using trace quantities of deuterium oxide. Biomed Mass Spectrom 1977;4:82–89.

11   Schoeller DA, van Santen E, Peterson DW, Dietz W, Jaspen J, Klein PD: Total body water measurements in humans with ^{18}O and ^{2}H labelled water. Am J Clin Nutr 1980;33:2686–2692.

12   Bland JM, Altman DG: Statistical methods for assessing agreement between two methods of clinical measurement. Lancet 1986;8:307–310.

13   Bell NA, McClure PD, Hill RJ, Davies PSW: Assessment of foot to foot bioelectrical impedance analysis for the prediction of total body water. Eur J Clin Nutr 1998;52:856–859.

Assoc. Prof. Peter S.W. Davies, School of Human Movement Studies, Faculty of Health,
Queensland University of Technology, Victoria Park Road, Kelvin Grove Qld 4059 (Australia)
Tel +61 7 3864 5830, Fax +61 7 3864 3980, E-Mail ps.davies@qut.edu.au

Jürimäe T, Hills AP (eds): Body Composition Assessment in Children and Adolescents.
Med Sport Sci. Basel, Karger, 2001, vol 44, pp 175–176

....

Conclusions and Perspectives

The fifteen papers that complete this monograph present a diversity of information relating to anthropometry and body composition in children and youth. The papers reflect the input of a selection of the top researchers from all over the world. The monograph presents new information about various methodological aspects and challenges in the measurement of body composition in young people. Almost without exception, contributors reinforce the viewpoint that the study of children, particularly where physical measurements are involved, is considerably more complicated compared with adults.

Several articles are presented about the measurement of body composition using the bioelectrical impedance (BIA) method. This is very understandable as the method is one of the simplest and more straightforward options and does not require very expensive equipment. Furthermore, it is relatively comfortable for the children who are measured. However, there is not universal consensus regarding the best approach to employ when utilising this method. For example, there is a need for more information about the influence of various anthropometric parameters on body resistance in prepubertal, pubertal and postpubertal children. These parameters need to be addressed in order to reduce the effects of inter-individual variance in resistance values, presumably related to differences in body size and shape. The lack of data is particularly pronounced in relation to the pubertal period when the most dramatic changes in the anthropometric profile of individuals occurs. Similarly, more specific equations for the calculation of different body composition parameters, including percent body fat and LBM, are needed. Potentially, we need corrections for each pubertal stage using, for example, the Tanner scale. There is also considerable merit in more widespread exploration of multi-frequency BIA machines and also segmental approaches to measurement. Similarly, there is a need to explore the use of different anthropometric parameters, especially girths, in body composition equations. Potentially, equations that utilise different anthropometric parameters and body resistance are more correct. On the one hand, we need new equations for the measurement of body composition in 'normal' schoolchildren, and on the other hand, we need equations for 'specific' groups such as the obese and particularly for young sportsmen. Some of the potential new horizons in these respects are addressed in this monograph.

In summary, this monograph provides answers to some of the questions related to the correct measurement of body composition in children. In the immediate future, the major challenge for researchers in the area will be to arrive at a consensus regarding the most appropriate methodologies to suit a range of settings and conditions (field or laboratory, simple or complicated) in the assessment of body composition in children. Much of the current software used in commercial equipment employs acceptable calibration equations that are used to derive body composition values. However, many such instruments lack suitable equations for children of different ages, gender and specific ethnic backgrounds. There are additional challenges for use of techniques in clinical settings and with sports populations.

Toivo Jürimäe, Tartu
Andrew P. Hills, Brisbane

Author Index

Subject Index

Breast development, anthropometric
  parameter relationships 80, 81

Cardiovascular disease (CVD), risk
  evaluation in adolescents using visceral
  adipose tissue
  anthropometric factors, variability 137, 138
  blood lipid profiles 134, 136, 137
  blood pressure measurement 134, 137
  overview 132
  statistical analysis 134, 135
Computed tomography (CT), body
  composition measurement 5

Densitometry, *see* Hydrostatic weighing
Dual-energy X-ray absorptiometry (DXA)
  accuracy, body composition
    measurement 5, 6
  advantages and disadvantages 5, 6, 10
  principle 5

Fat-free mass (FFM)
  body weight component 1
  children vs adults 2
  density 2, 3
  water fraction estimate 4
Fat mass (FM)
  body weight component 1
  density 2

Girth
  bioelectrical impedance analysis
    relationships at different measurement
    frequencies 64, 66, 69
  sexual maturation relationships, girls
    measurements 72
    outcomes 74, 76, 77, 82
    overview 71, 72
    statistical analysis 73
Gymnastics
  body image, females 139, 140
  prediction equation development, females
    anthropometry 140, 141, 149
    applications 151, 152
    bioelectrical impedance analysis
      141, 142, 149, 151, 152
    comparison of equations 144–146

external criteria 150, 151
performance tests and relationship
  with body composition
    143, 144, 147–149
skinfold equations 142, 143, 149–151
statistical analysis 144
subjects 140
somatotype, females 139, 148
training 139

Height, *see* Stature
Hydrostatic weighing
  bioelectrical impedance analysis reference
    method 48, 50
  overview, densitometry 3

Isotope dilution, total body water
  determination 3, 4, 169–172

Length
  bioelectrical impedance analysis
    relationships at different measurement
    frequencies 64, 69
  sexual maturation relationships, girls
    measurements 72
    outcomes 73, 74, 76, 78, 82
    overview 71, 72
    statistical analysis 73
LIPOMETER, *see* Subcutaneous adipose
  tissue topography (SAT-Top)

Magnetic resonance imaging (MRI)
  body composition measurement 4, 5
  visceral adipose tissue measurement
    132, 133, 135, 137

Near infra-red interactance method, body
  composition measurement 10

Obesity, *see also* Visceral adipose tissue
  (VAT)
  longitudinal relationship with eating and
    activity patterns in adolescence
    age changes, lifestyles 158
    body fat measurement 165
    dietary intake-physical activity
      relationships 160, 164, 165

Total body nitrogen (TBN)
  age relationship, children 27, 28, 30
  chemical maturity 30
  chronic disease effects, children 31–33
  direct vs indirect measurement
    26, 27
  neutron capture analysis
    measurement protocol 26, 27
    principle 25, 26
    prompt-gamma method 26, 33
  rationale for total body protein
    measurements 25
  regression equations, growth variables
    28–30
Total body potassium (TBK)
  age relationship, children 28
  measurement 4

Total body water (TBW), *see also*
  Bioelectrical impedance analysis (BIA)
  body weight component 1
  isotope dilution 3, 4, 169–172

Visceral adipose tissue (VAT)
  cardiovascular disease risk evaluation,
    adolescents
    anthropometric factors in variability
      137, 138
    blood lipid profiles 134, 136, 137
    blood pressure measurement 134, 137
    overview 132
    statistical analysis 134, 135
  correlation among measurement
    techniques 135, 137
  measurement 132, 133, 136
  prediction equations 132, 133, 137